THE
SMARTER
WAY

TO
EXERCISE • MOVE • EAT • THINK • LIVE

SUSAN FINLEY

Train**Smarter**
4225 Harpers Ferry Rd
Birmingham, AL 35213
www.wetrainsmarter.com
Printed in the United States of America

ISBN 978-1-7357098-0-2
ISBN 978-1-7357098-1-9

CONTENTS

NUTRITION

WEIGHT LOSS

BETTER HEALTH

MINDSET

INTRODUCTION

Every now and again, someone says something to me like, "I bet you were a cheer-leader (or gymnast or something else athletic)....." It astounds--and flatters--me because that couldn't be further from the truth.

The truth: The only team I ever got chosen for was the debate team.

I was smaller and younger than my classmates, the last chosen for teams in P.E. classes, but the first to look for if you needed homework to copy. My activities consisted of reading books, practicing piano, and watching TV. On weekends, my family might go "driving around." Our physical activity was exclusively doing chores. Movement wasn't about fun. It was about work.

It was the age of "labor saving devices" and everyone was looking to move less. We drank sweet tea and ate lots of white bread and fried chicken, okra, corn, and anything else we could fry.

Sooo.....when I was about 12 years old, I remember going to the pediatrician. I don't remember why we went, but I remember my mom being furious when we left the doctor's office. She was upset about a word he'd written on my chart. I felt so confused and discomforted about this word I'd never heard before and my mom's emotional reaction to it. I remember asking, "Mama, what does 'obese' mean?"

Thus began my decades-long preoccupation with weight loss. My parents managed their stress with food and we were all overweight. I saw the price my parents paid for our lifestyle. Mom had high blood pressure, high cholesterol, Type 2 diabetes, and ultimately needed both knees and shoulders replaced. Dad had back pain, stomach issues, Type 2 diabetes, and died WAY too young at 72.

Since my parents weren't physically active, I didn't get exposed to hiking, skiing, tennis, golf, bowling, or any recreational activity. We didn't even have access to a swimming pool. So I was a total misfit in physical education classes, which were suited to kids who were better coordinated, athletic and more comfortable in their body than I. Whenever possible, I got out of P.E by substituting other options, like "office aide," and was thrilled to discover I could substitute philosophy for the three quarters of physical education that Auburn required for graduation.

My first positive exercise experience was in Chapel Hill, NC, after my twins were born. My best friend convinced me to go to an exercise class with her and I went, despite having to peel a toddler off of each leg to get out of the house. Those classes were essentially calisthenics. The workouts were hard but going with a friend gave me the confidence and accountability to keep going. Later, I went to an aerobics studio with a name like "Total Woman" and discovered I felt much more energetic after going to these classes. Who knew that moving more could give you more energy?!

As I tried various exercise options, I discovered the amazing changes strength training could make. It's so empowering! At the same time, I was seeing my parents' health and their ability to do everyday things deteriorate.

I recognized that Dad's shoulder wouldn't have hurt if his back was stronger. Mom's knees wouldn't have gone bad and she wouldn't have had bunions if she'd had stronger hips. Her shoulders wouldn't have worn out if she'd had better posture and been stronger so her muscles could have supported her joints. Mom loved to go out, but for the last few years of her life, every outing was evaluated based on how many stairs were involved. I watched her world get more and more limited.

Knowing that exercise is critical to living well, I became downright evangelistic about saving people from the pain and disability I'd witnessed. Not only does exercise, particularly strength training, keep the body strong, it has the amazing effect of strengthening the mind, too. When you see what you're capable of doing, the self-confidence and self-sufficiency that result are life changing.

The world is full of people who don't know what they're missing. The average American walks only about a third of a mile a day and that includes walking around the house.

Why do so many people resist exercising? Most just don't know what to do. There's so much conflicting information—how do you know what to believe? They try high intensity workouts that leave them sore and injured so they think exercise is painful and quit. They sign up for a "6-Week Weight Loss Challenge" and either don't lose the weight or it's back in 6 more weeks.

So that program "didn't work" and they're off looking for something more effective, not understanding that weight is lost in the kitchen.

The people who have a special place in my heart are those who are like I was, who feel uncomfortable and awkward with exercise. Exercise doesn't have to be miserable and humiliating. You just have to find the right exercise fit. Once you start, it's all improvement from there. Success comes from developing a mindset of "progress over perfection" and committing to making exercise an essential part of your life. It's the best thing you can do for yourself. This kind of self-care can even mean the difference between life and death.

My goal with this book is to help you cut through the myths and misinformation about exercise and wellness. Now more than ever, we need to cherish and nourish our health and the right exercise program, along with good nutrition, is the way to do it. No one should suffer pain and disability when the right exercise can prevent it. Even if doing all the right things doesn't add years to your life, you can bet it will add life to your years.

Fitness business coaches say that long-term goals like moving well and feeling great for a lifetime just don't motivate people. They believe that people are more interested in short term goals like weight loss or looking good for a reunion.

I'm here to challenge that belief, based on all the people I've met who dream of living life to its fullest. Being strong and fit makes it possible to chase after kids and grandkids, avoid medications and their side effects, travel and sight-see without being exhausted, carry your groceries in one trip, and generally feel younger than your years.

I want everyone to see that they can create a life they love--a life without limits!

EXERCISE

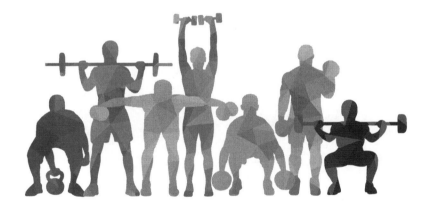

WHAT WE NEED IS A GOOD DOSE OF EXERCISE!

"How long will I have to do this?" The question caught me off-guard. My client had just finished a set and was taking a break.

I asked, "Do what? This exercise?"

"No, how long will I have to exercise?"

Taken aback by the question, I answered, "Only as long as you want to be healthy and feel young."

The failed resolution to work out and get in shape is a cliché despite the fact that the benefits of exercise could make a drug company rich beyond imagination if it could manufacture a drug that delivers the benefits of exercise without the side effects of medications.

Consider what exercise can do:

- Stop sarcopenia—the inevitable loss of muscle mass as we age
- Boost metabolic rate
- Moderate blood sugar
- Reduce blood pressure
- Increase "good" cholesterol
- Maintain joint integrity
- Alleviate stress and depression
- Improve posture and appearance

- Strengthen the immune system

- Contribute to the prevention of some cancers

- Increase strength, leading to greater levels of self-sufficiency and confidence

- Maintain balance and thinking skills as you age

Exercise has been called the closest thing we will ever have to the Fountain of Youth. Why is it so hard to motivate people to exercise? Certainly, there's a learning curve that can be intimidating.

But the greatest benefits accrue to those who go from doing nothing to doing something.

Making small changes is the name of the game.

I like to think of exercise the same way yogis approach their yoga practice—it's something you expect to do for the long haul. There's no "finish line" and no reason to do it at an intensity level that makes you miserable.

Embrace the idea that exercise is a way to take care of your body and amounts to preventive medicine.

Remember that you're making a commitment for a lifetime so even if your exercise program gets derailed occasionally, it's never too late to get back on the road of your fitness journey.

Exercise is the most powerful medicine the world has ever known…without the side effects!

A NEW WAY TO LOOK AT EXERCISING

Remember when Lance Armstrong was a hero?

Back then, I was so impressed that someone could, apparently, love riding excruciatingly long distances and punishing hills for hours on end, day after day.

Then, right before one of the Tours, I read a profile of him in The New Yorker, in which he said he didn't love those rides. He actually hated them! But he had that *goal*.....

You might think most people exercise because they just *love* it. **WRONG!**

I've had people look at me with admiration and ask, "Do you run every day?"

Heck, no. And lots of miles (and 3 marathons later) I still wouldn't tell you I love running. I do it because I think it's *worth* it.

Many mornings I've gotten up and thought I just didn't have it in me to do the run. So, I made a deal with myself....

I found a point half a mile from my house. I negotiated with myself to run that far on days I didn't think I felt like it. If I didn't feel better by the time I reached that point, I gave myself permission to turn around and go back home. At least I would have run a mile. But if I started feeling more energetic by that point, I kept going.

And most mornings, that was the case.

Just last week, I wasn't sure I was feeling rested enough to go but when I did, I felt so *good* when I got back and was glad I'd tried.

Sometimes life is especially stressful and exercise is a form of stress for your body. So, there will be times that you think you just can't do it.

But as I say when a client looks askance at a heavy weight, "You never know till you try!"

I spend all day around exercise equipment, but I struggle to make time for my own workouts. Summertime is especially hard for me to get motivated because I find it so depressing.

But I want to stay strong, healthy, self-sufficient, and pain-free, so I find a way to get a couple of workouts in, even if it's minimal.

Don't have time to get in a full workout? Give yourself *extra* credit if you make time to do part of one.

Don't let "perfect" get in the way of "good."

It took a lot of years for this Virgo to learn that lesson.

THE EXERCISE PYRAMID
A GUIDE TO EXERCISE CHOICES

Sometimes in your life you can dial down and make exercise a major part of your life. Other times you have to fit it in as best you can. But there's nothing to gain and everything to lose if you quit altogether, because there'll never be a perfect time.

What if you only have time for the barest minimum--what should be your priority?

I imagine an "Exercise Pyramid" in which you focus on the "base" and move up the pyramid as you have more time or interest.

An *appropriately designed* strength-training program is the base--the minimum that everyone should do.

Strength training

- keeps you strong and self-sufficient

- improves posture

- prevents joint pain

- alleviates stress and depression

- improves flexibility

- increases bone density

- improves balance

- boosts metabolic rate

- leads to greater self-sufficiency and confidence

- improves cardiovascular health

We're talking real strength training here--2-3 sets of 10-12 repetitions that are hard enough that you couldn't do more with good form. And while 2-3 times a week would be great, you can get by on 1-2 times a week if that's all the time you have. ***Even one time a week beats nothing at all!***

Strength training will make you a better runner, walker, golfer, bowler, desk jockey.... **it just makes you better at LIFE.**

If you have more time, you can move up the pyramid to endurance training. Maybe you really love to run or walk or row or swim. Endurance training ("cardio") can reduce stress and keep your heart strong. But while it's possible to see cardio improvements from strength training (we see it a lot via our heart rate sensors), you don't get strength improvements from cardio, because there's no progressive resistance.

Moving up the pyramid...you've got a fair amount of time and you've covered your strength and cardio bases? Add yoga. You won't get cardio benefit from yoga and little strength improvement beyond a point because you've only got your body weight for resistance. It's not as well-balanced as strength training because there's no element of "pulling." But it strengthens stabilizers and improves balance, with a mindfulness element you might not find in strength training.

Got lots of time and looking for something to do every day? Or maybe you used to take ballet and love dance exercise? Add Pilates, barre, or some form of dance. Dance is great for cardio and best of all, it has the elements of social connection and fun. That's worth a lot right there!

Just remember, doing anything beats doing nothing so when in doubt, keep moving!

THE 5 PILLARS OF MOVEMENT

We can thank Arnold Schwarzenegger and his bodybuilding pals for drawing attention to strength training back in the 1970's. For a lot of years, all we knew about strength training was what we learned from bodybuilders.

Bodybuilding exercises addressed particular muscles, referred to as "isolating" a muscle. On "leg day" you might do exercises specifically for the quads, the hamstrings, calves, and even adductors. On "chest day" there were specific exercises targeting the "upper chest" and the "lower chest," the "inner chest" and the "outer chest."

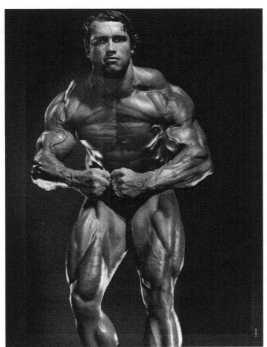

This was when the exercise machine market exploded. **Bodybuilders trained the bigger skeletal muscles and rarely any stabilizers, so it was perfect for them to have the machine hold the weight for them and all they had to do was move it.**

Over time, people realized that they didn't want to look like a bodybuilder--so why train like one? They wanted strong muscles, not necessarily big ones. It was the dawn of Functional Fitness Training.

Functional training focuses on movements, not individual muscles. You don't sit on a machine and let the machine stabilize the weight, you use your body's stabilizers. Rather than isolating muscles, your muscles learn to work optimally *together*.

We train according to Dan John's **5 Pillars of Movement:**

- Push—pushups, chest and overhead presses, Palloff presses
- Pull--pulling from all angles with a variety of hand positions
- Hinge--done on one or both legs, it will save your back & knees!
- Squat--a variety of squats, lunges, step-ups in various planes
- Loaded Carry--truly total body exercise

This training protocol prevents muscle imbalances, as we make sure we pull as much as we push. Movements on just one leg strengthen lower body stabilizers. Hinges and carries prevent back injuries by teaching good lifting and carrying technique.

There's also a 6th Pillar of "and then some" ground-based exercises that we consider to be critical, like side planks and mobility exercises.

Exercise prescription should be based on your goals. If you want big muscles, you need to train like Arnold. If you want to be strong, pain-free, and able to do what you want to do,....well, you need to train....smarter

TOP 4 MISTAKES PEOPLE MAKE WHEN STARTING A FITNESS PROGRAM AND HOW TO FIX THEM

According to Strava, the day most people are likely to give up on their New Year's resolution is January 19--they call it **"Quitter's Day."** Roughly 80% of people who make New Year's resolutions have dropped them by the second week of February.

Here are 4 ways that people get tripped up:

1. CHANGING TOO MANY HABITS AT ONCE

There's an 85% success rate adopting one new habit at a time. Trying to change two habits at once has a success rate of 35%. If you try to tackle 3 things at one time, your chances are virtually nil.

A more effective approach is **"The Goal Snowball."** Make a list of what you want to change, from easiest to hardest. Pick the easiest one and work on that for at least 2 weeks. Once that habit is established, move on to the next one.

Once you've mastered that one thing, build on it--"I'm going to start my dinners with a salad." Then build on that, "I'm going to start taking a walk after lunch (or dinner)." Over time these little changes "snowball" into major life changes.

My guru, Dan John says that when he is counseling someone on losing weight and getting fit, he starts with "Consciously drink 2 glasses of water a day." It seems ridiculously easy but little wins create a feeling of success and success encourages more success.

2. EXPECTING IMMEDIATE RESULTS

We're an "instant gratification" society and people approach change with the expectation that they'll see quick results. That's partly the fault of fitness pros who promise quick weight loss and overnight results.

The reality is, **exercising patience is the place to start.** Meaningful change is a marathon, not a sprint.

People lose patience and quit because the scale doesn't seem to budge or they don't see the changes they want to see right away. But lots of change happens that you can't see. Huge neurological changes are going on in the first weeks of an exercise program, while bones, tendons and ligaments are getting stronger.

Trust the system, be patient, and celebrate the successes. Little wins add up to big results *over time.*

3. NOT KNOWING YOUR "WHY"

Are you looking to increase your chances of living longer and better? Want to be able to do more with your kids/grandkids? Have a goal like participating in an active vacation?

Spend some time in self-reflection and ask yourself the 5 whys.1

Why do you want to exercise? To lose weight.

Why do you want to lose weight? Because I don't like the way I look.

Why don't you like the way you look? Because I'm 35 pounds overweight.

Why is losing 35 pounds important to you? Because I'm prediabetic, have low energy and I can't keep up with my kids anymore.

Why is keeping up with your kids important? Because they're young and I want to be a better parent to them for as long as possible.

4. TRYING TO GO IT ALONE

People start out fired up and then get side-lined by injury, work issues, family complications, and countless other factors.

Rather than letting it derail you completely, know that sometimes things just come up. Focus on your plans to get back to it as soon as possible.

Some people do better with an "accountabilibuddy." Some need trustworthy nutrition guidance. And most people need some exercise coaching. There's so much to know and a world of faulty information out there.

So get a coach. Even we coaches have coaches. It saves so much time and frustration, and dramatically increases the chance you'll reach your goals.

The only way to fail is to quit. And you're no quitter, right?

"WHY WEIGHT TRAINING IS RIDICULOUSLY GOOD FOR YOU"

Having been in the fitness industry for over 30 years, I've learned that without a doubt, strength training is the greatest game changer for your health and quality of life.

Time magazine agrees in "Why Weight Training Is Ridiculously Good For You."1

"Modern exercise science shows that **working with weights...may be the best exercise for lifelong physical function and fitness. '...resistance training is the most important form of training for overall health and wellness',** says Brad Schoenfeld, an assistant professor of exercise science at New York City's Lehman College...

- **It strengthens muscles, bones, tendons, and ligaments**

Many people think of weight training as exercise that augments muscle size and strength... But... the "load" that this form of training puts on bones and their supporting muscles, tendons and ligaments is probably a bigger deal when it comes to health and physical function....

... later in life, bone tissue losses accelerate and outpace the creation of new bone. That acceleration is especially pronounced among people who are sedentary and women who have reached or passed menopause... *This loss of bone tissue leads to the weakness and postural problems that plague many older adults.*

Resistance training counteracts all those bone losses and postural deficits" ... resistance training is really the best way to maintain and enhance total-body bone strength.

- **It improves blood sugar regulation, cholesterol levels, and blood pressure.**

During a bout of resistance training, your muscles are rapidly using glucose, and this energy consumption continues even after you've finished exercising. For anyone at risk for metabolic conditions—type-2 diabetes, but also high blood pressure, unhealthy cholesterol levels and other symptoms of metabolic syndrome—strength training is among the most-effective remedies, ...

- **It reduces inflammation--a major risk factor for heart disease and cancer**

... study from Mayo Clinic found that when overweight women did twice-weekly resistance training sessions, they had significant drops in several markers of inflammation.

- **It has tremendous psychological benefits**

More research has linked strength training to improved focus and cognitive function, better balance, less anxiety and greater well-being.

- **Maintaining strength later in life seems to be one of the best predictors of survival**

When we add strength...almost every health outcome improves. It used to be we thought of strength training as something for athletes, but now we recognize it as a seminal part of general health and well-being at all ages."

Most of all, it makes you *useful*.

Brian Johnson writes 2

"If we want to be a protector and hero to those around us, we need to focus on BEING USEFUL...

'Exercise only with the intention to carry out a physical gain or to triumph over competitors,' [Georges] Hébert believed, 'is brutally egoistic.' ... Hébert, consequently, came up with the strangest mission statement ever devised for getting in shape. He called it Méthode Naturelle—the Natural Method—and it would be ruled by a five-word credo that had zero to do with getting ripped, getting thin, or going for gold. In fact, it had zero to do with 'getting' anything; Hébert was heading the opposite direction.

'Etre fort pour etre utile,' Hébert declared. 'Be fit to be useful.' It was brilliant, really. Hébert came up with a complete philosophy for life...

No matter who you are, no matter what you're seeking or hope to leave behind after your time on the planet—is there any better approach than simply to be useful?

'Here is the great duty of man to himself, to his family, to his homeland and to humanity. *Only the strong will prove useful in difficult circumstances of life.'*'

Now, aren't you glad you lift weights? And if you don't, what are you waiting for?

THE PROBLEM WITH
"THE PAUSE-BUTTON MENTALITY"

Have you ever found yourself planning to start a diet on Monday, waiting to start an exercise program until after the holidays or thinking you'd start to take better care of yourself once the kids go back to school?

The folks at *Precision Nutrition* refer to that as "The Pause Button Mentality." 1

"I think it's normal — even commendable — to want to do your best. To consider taking time to regroup and then resume (or start over) when life feels easier…. this completely natural and well-meaning impulse is one of the fastest, surest, most reliable ways to sabotage your plans for improved nutrition, health, and fitness.

Starting fresh after you lose your way is a really comforting thought. That's probably why New Year's resolutions are so popular, especially following the indulgence-fueled holiday season. Give me that cheesecake. I'll pick my diet back up on Monday!… But here's the problem: The pause-button mentality only builds the skill of pausing…. This perceived relief is compounded by the illusion that *if we "start fresh" later we can find the magical "right time" to begin.*

It can feel absurd to try to improve your eating and exercise habits while you're in the midst of chronic stress / looking for a job / starting a new job / going on vacation / caring for aging parents / raising small children. **That's probably why there are so many 21-days this and 90-days that… But what do these intense fitness sprints teach you? The skill of getting fit within a very short (and completely non-representative) period of your life. What don't they teach**

you? The skill of getting fit (or staying fit) in the midst of a normal, complicated, "how it really is" sort of life.

It's not about willpower. It's about skills. In most fitness scenarios, you learn how to get fit under weird, tightly-controlled, white-knuckle life situations.... What you don't build is the ability to get fit under real-life conditions. That's why it doesn't stick...the natural and predictable consequence of having a limited skill set is short-term progress followed immediately by long-term frustration. What will be different next time?

...when our clients ask to press pause, we usually ask them: "What will be different when you come back?" Nine times out of 10, the honest answer is nothing. Nothing will be different. Life is just... happening. And it'll happen again in January, or after the baby is born, or after Mom gets better, or at any other arbitrary point you pick. And what then?

...There's never going to be a moment when things are magically easier. You can't escape work, personal, and family demands. Nor can you escape the need for health and fitness in your life.... you can't stop showing up for work and expect not to get fired. Or "take a break" from being married and not wind up divorced.... **Sometimes we're superstars. Most of the time we just do our best. We muddle through. We keep going. So, why do we expect it to be any different with fitness?**

Nowadays I like to think of my fitness and nutrition efforts as a dial. There are times when I want to dial my efforts up, and times when I want to dial them down. **But I never want to turn the dial off completely.**

... remember your new mantra... "Always something."

Perfection never happens in real life. We're always going to be doing the best we can with what we have. And that's okay.

We can still make progress toward our goals and still improve our health and our fitness — whatever's going on in our lives.

That progress doesn't happen if you "press pause" and wait for a better time."

Instead of turning your habits on or off, think of them as a dial that you turn up when you can, and turn down when you have to. Consider the spectrum:

Movement

1. Park farther from the office to walk more
2. Take stairs instead of elevator
3. 10 minute workout next to bed in the morning
4. Reasonably challenging 30 minute workout 3x/week
5. 3-30 minute workouts/week + daily 20 minute walk
6. 3-1 hour gym workouts/week + daily walk
7. Gym routine 4x/week, hike on weekends
8. 5-1-hour workouts' week + daily 1 hour walk
9. Challenging 60-90 minute workout 6x/week

Nutrition

1. Replace 1 meal with less processed one
2. Add side salad to your lunch
3. Try 1 new healthy recipe/week
4. Sit at table for most meals
5. Protein with each meal
6. Protein + portion of fruit or vegetable at most meals
7. Prep food for week in advance; 6 servings of vegetables/day
8. Prep food in advance, protein + vegetables at each meal
9. Eat mostly local, plan all meals in advance, each "perfectly" balanced

Overall Wellness

1. 5 minutes of wind-down time before bed
2. 5 minutes to plan for the next day's workouts/nutrition
3. Regular 5 minute breaks from work for fresh air and sunlight
4. Turn off electronics 30 minutes before bed; read book and chill out
5. Daily walk outdoors with loved one; pet your dog

6. 1 massage/month; hug a loved one

7. 10 minute meditation/day; 7 hours sleep/night; hugs

8. Do something nice for others; engaging hobby; minimal screen time

9. Fulfilling paid/volunteer work; daily meditation; more sleep; express yourself

One of my favorite mantras is "**No Zero Days.**"

There will be times when getting a 1 in even one of these categories is the best you can do—maybe just one perfect pushup beside your bed—it's still progress toward taking care of yourself and reinforcing healthy habits.

And that won't happen if you keep hitting the "pause button!"

CAPTAIN MARVEL'S GOT NOTHING ON YOU!

One of the many benefits of strength training is how it makes people feel stronger *mentally*. Time and again I've seen people gain confidence and mental fortitude as a result of getting physically stronger.

Brie Larson--Captain Marvel--was a self-described[1]

> "introvert with asthma before this film, so I had a lot of work to do, and I just started to fall in love with it. I started to fall in love with the way my body was changing and transforming.....I just wanted to be a brain, so I've only cared about reading books and understanding words, and anything that involved my body made me itchy. But this was an opportunity for me to... make my body mine."

There's something empowering about getting stronger. You learn to get comfortable with trying things because strength training taught you "you don't know what you can do 'till you try."

You discover that you have the power to change your health, the power to feel better, the power to function better......***the power to decide who you become.***

Still, there are women who fear that getting stronger will make them "bulky" despite all the evidence to the contrary.

Brie's experience should allay those fears. Here's what she accomplished, as documented on Instagram:

- 215 pound deadlifts

- 10 Pullups

- 400-pound hip thrust

- Push-ups with 50 pounds of chains

- Pushing a Jeep up hill

This is what she looked like at the Captain Marvel Premiere:

Brie was just like the rest of us, never imagining what she was capable of accomplishing. She focused on the process, without worrying about the outcome.

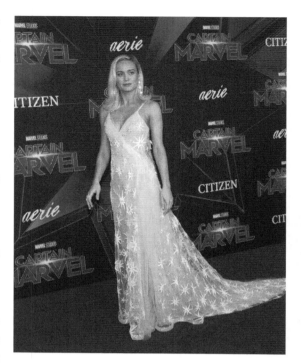

We can always be a work in progress, if we choose to be. Exercising leads to being stronger--mentally and physically. Better eating habits make us healthier. There will always be setbacks but step by step, consistent effort leads to *becoming who you want to be.*

You have the power!

STRETCHING DOESN'T WORK AND WHY SOME PEOPLE SHOULDN'T DO IT AT ALL

Clients often come in and sheepishly confess, "I never stretch...." To which I reply, "No worries. Neither do I."

Almost 20 years ago I happened upon a course at a personal training convention, never dreaming that this session was going to rock my world.

The presenter was Greg Roskopf, founder of Muscle Activation Techniques. I knew nothing about this course or what to expect. Greg strode into the room and announced, "I'm here to tell you that stretching doesn't work."

"What? That's ridiculous!" I thought, and considered all the hours I'd spent with books, classes, and videos about stretching. I was known as the "expert" on stretching and people often approached me saying, "(Fill in the blank) hurts. What do I need to stretch?"

Greg continued, "How many of you have clients who come in and you stretch and you give them stretches to do at home but they always stay tight in all those same places?"

Hands went up, including mine. "How many of you have clients who go to physical therapy, only to go back over and over again?" More hands were raised. "I'm telling you, **stretching doesn't work.**"

This was a seminal moment in my career. I have since taught Muscle Activation to all the fitness pros I have mentored and it has been a powerful tool in corrective exercise.

Muscle Activation teaches that if a muscle or muscle group appears to be "tight" it's because the opposing muscle or muscle group is weak or "inhibited" and doesn't effectively oppose the tight muscles. Stretching the tight muscle is ineffective because it will just spring back to where it was. There's nothing to hold it in place. But if you activate the weak side, it pulls the tight side back into place. As many clients can testify, it works like *magic*!

A classic complaint is "tight hamstrings." You may have seen someone lying on their back, pulling one leg up in the air. But "tight hamstrings" are a *symptom*, not the problem. The problem is tight *hip flexors*, resulting from sitting, overstriding, recreational activities like biking and golfing, and faulty posture.

The hip flexors pull the pelvis down in front, pulling on the hamstrings. The hamstrings aren't *tight*, they're *taut*.

Muscle activation calls on the hip extensors (the glutes) to "wake up" and oppose the hip flexors so the pelvis can move back to neutral and reduce the pull on the hamstrings. Such imbalances cause issues in the shoulders, knees, hips, and back.

New franchises of "stretch clinics" have been opening up across the country. This stretching may feel good, but doesn't create lasting change, particularly *passive* stretching, in which one person stretches another.

Some people absolutely should not stretch.

Furthermore, don't stretch:

- **Before exercise**–Stretching before exercise *interferes* with athletic performance. Your body needs a certain level of tension to create power. Reconsider stretching before your run or workout. Joint mobility exercises pre-workout are a more effective practice.

- **Post injury**–There is *protective tension* around an area that has been injured. Stretching a previously injured area works against the healing process. Gentle movement is the recommended approach.

- **If you're hypermobile**–People who are hypermobile (aka "double-jointed") often stretch a lot, *despite the fact that they have inordinate ranges of motion.* Trigger points in their muscles send muscle tension messages to their brain, in an attempt to maintain joint stability--*protective tension.* **Hypermobile people need muscle tension for joint stability and should NOT stretch.**

- **Beyond normal range of motion**–I've checked range of motion in some people who say, "I can go back further than that." More range of motion is not better, beyond a point. That destabilizes the joint.

- **A muscle in spasm**–The most common cause of muscle spasm is a response to a muscle having been *overstretched*. That muscle spasm you have by your shoulder blade or the "crick in your neck" when you get up in the morning comes from the muscle spending too much time in a stretched position. Again, it needs gentle full-range motion.

- **Areas that are already overstretched**–such as the neck, hamstrings, and iliotibial band. Stretching these areas could cause a strain.

Focus on *joint mobility* rather than stretching. Address limited ranges of motion by strengthening areas lacking full range of motion.

Strengthening weak links alleviates all sorts of aches and pains and *a well-balanced strength training program effectively addresses issues that stretching simply doesn't.*

The question to ask isn't "What do I need to **stretch**...?" but "What do I need to **strengthen**...?"

JUMP SQUATS AND SILVER SNEAKERS

"I was calling to see if you offer PUH-LAH-TEE classes or classes for senior citizens."

That's a voicemail I received last week. I had to wonder if the woman who didn't know how to pronounce Pilates knew what she was asking for--and I wondered the same thing about "senior citizen classes."

What is a senior citizens' class? Why is it different from any other class? Does it reflect an expectation that old people are incapable of doing what young people do? It got me thinking about expectations......

I see coaches expect less of people of a certain age, especially if they're women.

I see people expect less of themselves because they've reached a certain age.

And I hear a lot of expectation that the future inevitably leads to disability.

But I see *ability* and not *age*.

I've worked with lots of 30 and 40 year olds who are weak, have faulty alignment and are certainly unfit. And I know 70 year olds who are strong and capable of doing anything they want to do.

If I told you we were going to visit a room full of 6 year olds, you'd expect to see a room full of people who look very similar. But a room full of 60 year olds could look wildly diverse!

A quality coaching program takes into consideration abilities and limitations and these factors aren't determined simply by the number of birthdays you've celebrated.

As we get older, typically we become less active. So we lose muscle, not so much because of age as lack of use.

Ever wonder why it's said that having children later in life keeps you young? It's because those older parents are chasing toddlers, while parents who got an earlier start are sitting at dance recitals and athletic events. Those sedentary practices easily become habits.

The big thing that people lose as they get older is their Type 2 muscle fibers--the **power** fibers. Use it or lose it, they atrophy from lack of use. But they're critical to the ability to react quickly--sprint to grab a child who's headed for the street, jump out of someone's way, catch yourself if you lose your balance, or hoist a heavy weight--maybe just that delivery from Amazon!.

Many physiologists now recommend explosive exercise for people of ALL ages, especially those over 40.

The Wall Street Journal recently ran an article on the "Best Exercises for Your 50s, 60s, 70s And Beyond."1

Here are some of the exercises:

1. 50s–Jump Squats, Side Planks, Lunge Jumps, Overhead Push-Presses
2. 60s–Squats, Lunges, Burpees, Dumbbell Curl and Press
3. 70s–Bulgarian Split Squats, Kettlebell Swings, Standing Windmills
4. 80s–Squats, Lunges, Lying Windmills–we love these!

That's how **we** train "senior citizens!"

So, I'm challenging you to expect that you can accomplish whatever you set your mind to do.

Age doesn't define who you are--it's simply the number of years the world has had to enjoy your presence!

YOU DON'T HAVE TO RUN FAR–OR FAST–TO LIVE LONGER

There's good news for the time-crunched, who feel they don't have time for the 75 minutes of vigorous aerobic exercise each week that federal guidelines recommend and only about half of Americans do. According to *Time* magazine1

> "In an analysis of 14 studies, researchers tracked deaths among more than 232,000 people from the U.S., Denmark, the U.K. and China over at least five years.... **People who said they ran any amount were less likely to die during the follow-up than those who didn't run at all. Runners were 27% less likely to die for any reason, compared with nonrunners, and had a 30% and 23% lower risk of dying from cardiovascular disease and cancer, respectively. This was true even for those who didn't log a great deal of time.**

> 'Regardless of how much you run, you can expect such benefits,' says Zeljko Pedisic, associate professor at the Institute for Health and Sport at Victoria University in Australia, and one of the authors of the new analysis...

> 'The physical demands of running affect just about every system of the body in a beneficial way.... Take the cardiovascular system. Running forces it to adapt by 'generating more capacity,' ... You grow more capillaries and small arteries, and that helps lower your blood pressure.' Running is good at guarding against cancer partly because it uses up blood sugar, starving the cancer cells that rely on it for fuel. And it protects you in other ways not necessarily measured in the latest research: by decreasing inflammation, for example, which is at the root of many diseases, and stimulating the production of a pro-

tein that improves brain health…'Vigorous physical activity has been shown to be by far—with no close second—the best way to prevent Alzheimer's,' he notes."

Possibly the best news is that **there was no additional advantage to running more than 50 minutes per week or how fast you run.**

Read that again--50 minutes a WEEK! And it doesn't matter how fast you run.

> "…people run for life-giving reasons, not just death-defying ones. 'Mortality is an important variable to think about, but there's also illness, and happiness, and vitality,' … 'Some people are running in order to stave off Alzheimer's, and other people to prevent heart disease, and other people because it makes them feel better and others for depression.'"

But one finding is clear: anything greater than zero MPH is where you'll reap the biggest benefits.

What about injuries? Will running will destroy your knees? More good news!2

> "… a recent small study found that **30 minutes of running actually lowered inflammation in runners' knee joints, leading many to question whether running really does increase a person's risk for injuries—or if it helps prevent them.**
>
> The researchers expected to find an increase in molecules that spur inflammation in people's knee fluid after they ran, but they didn't. Instead, they found that pro-inflammatory markers actually decreased after a 30-minute run.
>
> ..this suggests that there is probably an evolutionary advantage to allow us to run relatively short distances where our bodies protect cartilage from damage by decreasing inflammation…Long distance running may result in a situation where overwhelming the knee's ability to decrease inflammation occurs, leading to the potential for joint degeneration."

Like so many things, there appears to be a dose response to running. Some is great. More isn't necessarily better. Too much is…well, you know…

NEAT—THE NON-EXERCISE
WAY TO EXERCISE

Have you ever known anyone who "can't sit still"? Even when they're sitting, they're fidgeting.

That fidgeting is an example of **NEAT**--*Non–Exercise Activity Thermogenesis*--daily activities that don't include sleep and exercising. Little movements, like walking around instead of sitting, moving every hour, taking the stairs instead of the elevator... offset the effect of a generally sedentary lifestyle.

Research shows that sitting less and moving more leads to living longer. But *getting an hour's workout during the day has not proven to counteract the effect of sitting the rest of the day.1*

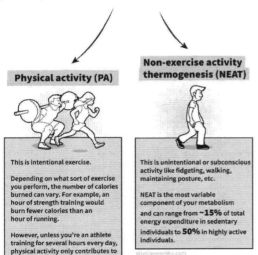

Physical activity (PA)

This is intentional exercise.

Depending on what sort of exercise you perform, the number of calories burned can vary. For example, an hour of strength training would burn fewer calories than an hour of running.

However, unless you're an athlete training for several hours every day, physical activity only contributes to about **10-15%** of total energy expenditure.

Non-exercise activity thermogenesis (NEAT)

This is unintentional or subconscious activity like fidgeting, walking, maintaining posture, etc.

NEAT is the most variable component of your metabolism and can range from **~15%** of total energy expenditure in sedentary individuals to **50%** in highly active individuals.

physiqonomics.com

"Certain markers for inflammation have been found to increase when NEAT is not a regular part of your day.... Researchers have seen C-reactive protein related to inflammation, triglycerides, and blood sugar increases in those who don't achieve NEAT on a regular basis. Heart health for those not achieving NEAT throughout the day is concerning...inactivity for just one day can cause cell processes to fail, allowing the breakdown of fats in the blood. This, in turn, lowers good cholesterol (HDL). ***Small movements throughout the day add up, and the cumulative effect is an increased metabolic rate....*** Sedentary jobs lead to lower levels of NEAT. NEAT could be the difference between gaining or losing weight, due to the accumulation of energy throughout the day. Instead of getting the average sedentary time for Americans at a whopping nine to ten hours per day, get up and move around more often. Whether you're gardening, taking a lap around the office, or even standing up during your conference calls—it all counts. The main thing is that you stay moving more than you sit still for your overall health."2

HOW MUCH NEAT DO I NEED?

There are no official rules but **adding a total of about two and a half hours of standing and light walking around the house or office** should do it. My Fitbit reminds me to get 250 steps every hour.

HOW CAN YOU INCREASE YOUR NEAT?

- Take the stairs whenever possible.
- Set a goal of getting at least 250 steps every hour during the day.
- Stand up and move around when you're on the phone.
- Park a little further from your destination.
- Meet friends to walk, instead of sitting at a bar or coffeeshop.
- Take the dog for walks.
- Park the car and go inside, rather than using a drive-through.
- Make multiple trips to carry in the groceries, instead of carrying the whole car load at one time.

ONE THING YOU PROBABLY CAN'T DO?

Become a fidgeter, if you're not already "wired" to be one. But that's ok, just take a walk instead.

Now, if you'll excuse me, I need to crank up my NEAT....

"IT MUST BE TRUE—I READ IT ON THE INTERNET..."

It is so frustrating as a fitness professional, to see health and fitness misinformation being disseminated to the public, who likely won't know any better.

I took one well-known magazine to task recently for their story about how to burn more calories and strengthen muscles with *walking*.

Strength training is a completely different energy system with completely different protocols from endurance work. Exercise doesn't burn a lot of calories and exercising shouldn't be focused on losing weight.

The magazine's editors didn't seem to be especially grateful for being set straight.....

Apparently, they aren't the only ones who aren't keeping current because my email from another mainstream health publication asked today, "What's the Best Exercise to Lose Weight: Cardio or Lifting Weights?"

That's a ridiculous question to ask. Exercise is unequaled for its benefit for SO many things but it's not the best approach to weight loss. It shouldn't be an "either/or" proposition. At the **end** of the article they finally mention...

> "It's also important to remember one essential fact about exercise and weight loss, says Slentz. **'Exercise by itself will not lead to big weight loss. What and how much you eat has a far greater impact on how much weight you lose,'** he says. That's because it's far easier to take in less energy (calories) than it is to burn significant amounts and it's very easy to cancel out the few hundred calories you've burned working out with just one snack."

They go on to say, "For the biggest fitness gain/weight loss bang for your exercise buck, combine the two..."

I'm nodding along with this one, (though you can't effectively "combine the two") and then they blow it with...

> "...doing your strength training first and finishing off with your cardio. An American Council on Exercise study on exercise sequencing found that your heart rate is higher—by about 12 beats per minute—during your cardio bout when you've lifted weights beforehand. That means more calories burned."

Actually, it probably means that the cardio is harder and takes more effort—hence the higher heart rate—because the muscles are tired. *That has nothing to do with the calorie burn.* A run outside in the heat may feel really hard but it doesn't mean you burn more calories than you would on a beautiful fall day.

A **higher heart rate does not mean you're burning more calories.** That's like saying you'll burn more calories watching *Cape Fear* (ever see this movie? I'll never forget how my heart was pounding) than watching the *British Bake Off.* Or that if I get my heart rate up by drinking caffeine before a run I'll burn more calories. Wrong, wrong, wrong.

You can raise your heart rate by using small muscles to wave your arms around--which is one theory about why orchestra conductors live so long. Or you could run or walk and get your heart rate to that same level.

Which do you think burns more calories?

Obviously, moving your body weight through space using big muscles.

You know more than a health magazine writer!

Don't believe everything you read...except what you see here!

FLEXIBILITY IS NO LONGER A PRIORITY

A lot of clients come in worried about their lack of "flexibility" and think they need to do more stretching. You already know how I feel about that, but my opinion is going mainstream.

Sports Medicine journal has published an article, "The Case for Retiring Flexibility as a Major Component of Physical Fitness," in which a researcher says,

> "The current paper proposes flexibility be retired as a major component of physical fitness, and consequently, stretching be de-emphasized as a standard component of exercise prescriptions for most populations. First, I show flexibility has little predictive or concurrent validity with health and performance outcomes (e.g. mortality, falls, occupational performance) in apparently healthy individuals, particularly when viewed in light of the other major components of fitness (i.e., body composition, cardiovascular endurance, muscle endurance, muscle strength). Second, I explain that *if flexibility requires improvement, this does not necessitate a prescription of stretching in most populations. Flexibility can be maintained or improved by exercise modalities that cause more robust health benefits than stretching (e.g., resistance training)."*

YES! Read that again: **"Flexibility can be maintained or improved by exercise modalities that cause more robust health benefits than stretching (e.g., resistance training)."**

That's exactly what we have learned from replacing stretching with balanced strength training programs.

He goes on to say that deleting stretching from fitness protocols will increase efficiency and testing accuracy.

> "Retirement of flexibility as a major component of physical fitness will simplify fitness batteries; save time and resources dedicated to flexibility instruction, measurement, and evaluation; and prevent erroneous conclusions about fitness status when interpreting flexibility scores."

Stretching before exercise or competition has been proven to impede sports performance. To that point, he says,

> "De-emphasis of stretching in exercise prescriptions will ensure stretching does not negatively impact other exercise and does not take away from time that could be allocated to training activities that have more robust health and performance benefits."

Mobility exercises have proven to be significantly more effective than stretching. They actually create change because they strengthen weaker muscles rather than yanking on the tighter muscles.

Some people just like the way stretching feels. It's fair to say there might be some *psychological* benefit from it, but its *physiological* benefits are highly overrated.

Stretch if you think it feels good (unless you're hypermobile--then **DON'T!**).

A PICTURE IS WORTH 1000 WORDS

About 30 years ago, I came across this photo in a research article by William Evans from Tufts University. Pretty amazing, right?

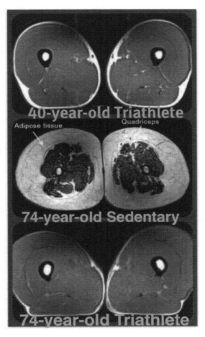

The solid white part in the middle is the thigh bone, surrounded by muscle. The white part around the edge is fat. Notice the loss of muscle and amount of fat in the leg of the sedentary man.

We start to lose muscle around the age of 30 and continue to lose, on average, 10% per decade. We generally think of people as getting old and frail, when actually, they're getting old and weak.

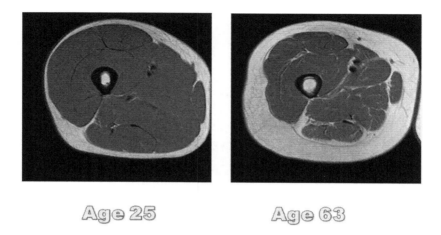

Age 25   Age 63

Strength training can stop this loss of muscle, known as "sarcopenia," and keep bones strong, as well. **I've had clients improve from osteopenia and the beginning stage of osteoporosis to normal levels of bone density just from strength training and becoming more active.**

Maintaining muscle mass is important for...

- Weight management. It takes additional calories to sustain muscle.

- Longer life. The more muscle, the longer you live, according to a long-term study published in the American Journal of Medicine.

- Preventing diabetes. Muscle tissue removes glucose from the bloodstream. The more muscle you have, the less predisposed you are to develop diseases such as diabetes.

- Lower injury risk. Being strong prevents injuries from doing everyday things like picking up kids or working in the yard. In addition, muscles protect our joints and bones against breaks and dislocations. Since tendons and cartilage grow stronger with our muscles, we become less susceptible to sprains and tears.

- Improved mood. Scientists at Sweden's Karolinska Institute ran a series of tests on mice and found that muscle removes a substance that accumulates in the blood during stress. Mice with greater skeletal muscle were less susceptible to depression--in fact, they weren't susceptible at all!

- Increased immunity. Muscle tissue is the only place that the body can store amino acids, so it plays a huge role in strengthening our immune system. Amino acids (such as glutamine, arginine and cysteine) are important to our ability to respond to pathogens and other toxic compounds in the body. The smaller our muscles, the smaller our amino acid stores and the less able we are to fight off disease and infections.

It's a "use it or lose it" proposition and muscle mass is something we can't afford to lose!

WHEN EXERCISE IS A MATTER OF LIFE OR DEATH

Of all the dozens of benefits of exercise, there's one I'd never thought about.

Erik Fredrickson talks about being diagnosed with leukemia at the age of 35.1

> "....even as vulnerable as I felt, I had something powerful on my side. My level and experience with exercise had not only strengthened me physically prior to the diagnosis but I noticed that *it influenced the way my doctors viewed and handled my treatment. As a result, I had reassurance during the rigors ahead and my immune system had a head start on the comeback it was about to make.*"

And come back he did. He did a 150 mile bike ride. Then he followed that up with an 18 mile paddleboard charity event.

Last year, 5 years after his initial diagnosis, he was again diagnosed with leukemia.

> "I haven't personally met a doctor (and I've met many) that didn't agree that my *"fitness" played a key role in aiding me through treatment or the ability to recover from its side effects.* I knew this "strength" helped me in so many ways and continues to create momentum for my recovery moving forward. **I didn't rely on exercise for prevention; I use it as a weapon that's in my power to wield to help face any adversity.**"

What if your fitness influenced your doctors' decisions?

> "Recently a good friend of mine in his eighties was diagnosed with cancer.... While we were discussing some of the experiences we were

going through, he mentioned an interaction he had with his doctor. He was told **if he hadn't been in such good physical shape, they wouldn't have bothered to treat him. I was confirmed in my belief that the strength we earned from choosing to exercise, helped us get through our toughest times but may very well have saved his life.**

As I was writing this, my friend sent me a video of himself competing in a bench press competition at 85 years old. I can't express the inspiration and joy that I have for him.....**I once looked at exercise as a preventive activity that helped me look better and feel good. I later learned that one of the biggest benefits I never saw coming was that it may have given my friend a second chance at life...exercise fortified me to withstand cancer treatment, hastened my recovery and remains a weapon for any threats that may be around the corner."**

I've seen first-hand how a dire prognosis can come out of nowhere. Should that day come, you're far better prepared to deal with the illness and its treatment if you're strong and fit.

In fact, your fitness will affect how aggressively the doctors choose to treat your disease.

Maybe you know you "need to do something" but you don't know what to do or figure you'll get around to it someday.

Turns out, your life might just depend on it.

THE TRUTH--"CORE TRAINING" IS A MEANINGLESS TERM

A man recently broke "the plank world record" by holding a plank for over 8 hours.

That reflects a lot of mental toughness--but from a fitness perspective, it's about as worthwhile as seeing how many people you can stuff in a Volkswagen.

Somehow, "holding a plank" became synonymous with "core strength."

Can we agree to stop using the word, "core"? It's so broad, it's meaningless. The **core is technically everything from the shoulders to the knees.** Given the global aspect of the core, **most strength training exercises are core exercises.** When someone says, "My core is weak." do they mean shoulders? Glutes? Abdominals?

What most people are thinking when they say that, is that they think their abdominals are weak. How do they judge that? Because they don't have a flat belly? Because they heard it's the cause of their back pain?

Back pain does not mean your core is weak.

I don't know that I've ever come across anyone who had "a weak core," which is to say, their core was any weaker than the rest of their body.

There are *whole fitness classes* structured around "working the core." Ever hear of one for "working the shoulders" or "training for glute strength"?

The likely scenario is that **people don't have core strength issues, they have core timing issues.** Here's where the madness began:1

> "Professor Paul Hodges ... performed experiments by attaching electrodes to two groups of people, one with healthy backs and another with chronic back pain.... the healthy group engaged a deeply embedded muscle called the transversus abdominis, causing it to contract and support the spine just before movement. In those with back pain, no such engagement took place, leaving the spine less supported. Hodges then claimed that this muscle could be strengthened by "drawing in" the stomach during exercises and this provided some protection against back pain.
>
> What he failed to see was that this wasn't an issue of poor *strength,* but poor *coordination.* **Despite no clear link to core strength, the concept quickly spread spawning a huge rise in exercise classes ..... And before you knew it, a stable core was lauded as a prerequisite in the fight against back pain and postural problems.**
>
> Thomas Nesser, ... later tried to establish a positive link between core stability and the ability to perform ordinary daily tasks, but failed! He says that **'despite the emphasis fitness professionals have placed on functional movement and core training for increased performance, our results suggest otherwise.'** When he looked at top football players he found that those with a strong core played no better than those without. He concluded that **'the fitness industry took a piece of information and ran with it. The assumption of 'if a little is good, then more must be better' was applied to core training and it was completely blown out of proportion.'"**

If you're not using your core in almost every exercise you do, you're doing it wrong.

The trunk muscles are an integral part of most exercises--*they're team players*-- and don't need to be isolated.

Don't even get me started on "training the obliques"....

Planks are an ok exercise. Certainly, no gold standard and done poorly more often than not. If you can hold that plank more than 8 seconds, it's time to add additional challenges to it--TRX exercises are moving planks.

Think of the plank as your neutral alignment and learn how to move well from that position.

Life isn't lived isometrically.....unless you're gunning for a world record.

YOU NEVER NEED TO DO ANOTHER CRUNCH—UNLESS THIS IS YOUR GOAL

What exercises do you think of when you think about abdominal/core exercises?

Planks had their moment, but the quintessential abdominal exercises have been sit-ups and crunches.

Sit-ups fell out of favor when we realized that a full sit-up uses your hip flexors to pull you up. Hip flexors attach in the lumbar spine, and that's why people found that sit-ups hurt their back.

To make things worse, once the hip flexors get short and tight, they pull your pelvis forward, creating a potbelly.

Well, that's counterproductive!

Crunches replaced them--you don't sit all the way up, so you're much less likely to use your hip flexors, saving the stress on your back.

But it can be more stressful for the neck, due to holding up your head directly against gravity. People often pull on their neck as they're supporting their head. And crunches create a different kind of stress on the back--a lot of anterior spinal compression. (Visualize how they flatten out the curve of the low back.)

The body is able to tolerate some measure of compression but you never know when your back is going to lose its tolerance.

As exercise moved into a more functional realm, crunches didn't fit the standard of being a movement you use in daily living.

Crunches use the rectus abdominis.

Stabilizing the trunk for daily life requires coordination of the rectus abdominis, transverse abdominis, obliques, quadratus lumborum, a variety of hip muscles..... It makes more sense to exercise using the whole body to teach those muscles how to work well together.

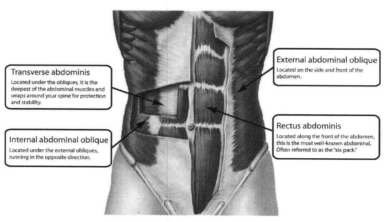

repkefitness.com

I can't say it enough, if you're not using your abdominal muscles in every exercise you do, you're doing them wrong.

WHO SHOULD BE DOING CRUNCHES?

Crunches are an effective tool for bodybuilders and physique competitors who are looking to develop the appearance of their "6-pack." They are trying to increase the *size* of those muscles, best done by adding load to the exercise.

Then at competition time, they use extreme dieting to keep a layer of fat from obscuring the muscles.

If you're thinking that you'd like the 6-pack, just not the dieting, think again.

First, the muscles will never be visible as long as there's a layer of fat over them--and getting that lean takes a lot of effort.

Second, if you build the muscles and don't lose the fat, you develop a thicker midsection, something that most people are trying to avoid.

NOT LOOKING TO SHOW OFF YOUR ABS?

You can get strong, functional abdominals with great exercises like straight arm pull-downs, pullovers, bus drivers, and a world of other exercises that won't hurt your neck and back.

These exercises not only keep your abdominals strong, they teach you how to use them in concert with a lot of other muscles...the way they work best.

ARE YOUR MUSCLES CONFUSED? THE PART "MUSCLE CONFUSION" PLAYS IN YOUR WORKOUTS

Back in the early bodybuilding days, Joe Weider, father of bodybuilding, created certain principles, one of which was "muscle confusion." The idea was that workouts need to change frequently because muscles would get used to the same exercises and then stop adapting.

If you ever did P90X workouts, you've heard of it.

More recently, that concept has been questioned by people who say that most exercisers have too *much variety.* They believe that always changing exercises and workouts leads to not becoming more proficient or getting stronger in the individual exercises.

The *New York Times* reported a new study, which was published in *PLOS One*, in which a group of researchers tested the impact of muscle confusion.1

They divided volunteers into two groups. One performed standard exercises in the same order four days a week, increasing weight loads as the exercises got easier.

The other group did the same number of exercises and lifted roughly the same amount of weight but used a special app that created a different workout each session, from a database of 80 exercises.

After 8 weeks, the volunteers were evaluated and researchers then compared results and found that **gains in muscular size and strength were almost exactly the same,** whether they had maintained the same routines or often switched them up.

BUT...the volunteers who participated in the varied workouts reported greater motivation to work out. **The biggest difference was mental!**

This research confirms the approach we take at Train**Smarter**. Workouts are based on the fundamental pillars of push, pull, hinge, squat, and loaded carry. But we use different variations of those movements.

If you want to get better at a particular exercise, say the bench press, then you should do more bench pressing.

But most people want to get stronger at LIFE. And that involves a lot of different kinds of movement.

There are so many things that can get in the way of exercising. If we can make it more interesting...dare I say *fun?*...then we've got a win all around!

HOW ACCURATE ARE CALORIE COUNTS FROM GYM EQUIPMENT AND FITNESS TRACKERS?

Recently a client was telling me about his elliptical workout, "I burned over 500 calories!"

All together now: **Exercise isn't about burning calories.** And you can't trust the calorie burn the machine tells you.

The number of calories you burn in any activity is affected by your

- height
- weight
- muscle mass
- fitness level
- level of stress
- sleep quality
- hormones
- and lots of other things....

From *Nutrition Action*: 1

> "Trying to determine how many calories somebody is burning is not easy," says John Porcari, professor of exercise and sport science at the University of Wisconsin–La Crosse. Porcari writes the calorie-burn equations for some companies that make exercise machines.

"First, the more work you do, the more calories you burn," notes Porcari. (Work is the amount of effort you exert and for how long.)

"Second, a bigger person burns more calories because they have more body to move. If a machine doesn't consider body weight, you have to question how accurate it is."

Machines also can't control for other factors. For example:

Fitness level. "Beginners often have more extraneous movements than seasoned exercisers, so they burn more calories doing the same activity," says Porcari.

Kinda like me in the swimming pool…

Handrails. If you hold on to the rails on a treadmill or stair climber, you burn fewer calories.

Walking or jogging? You burn more calories per minute when jogging than walking, but a treadmill can't tell if you're walking fast or jogging slowly.

Ellipticals are the trickiest. "…ellipticals have a fixed stride length, so if I'm really short, I have to do more work than someone who is taller."

How far off are most machines? "They may be as much as 20 to 30% high or low," says Porcari. So if you burned 300 calories, your bike may say anywhere from 210 to 390 calories.

What about Fitbits, Garmins, Apple Watches, and other fitness trackers?

"Their calorie estimates are often worthless," says Porcari. "Some try to quantify how much work you're doing based on your heart rate, your speed, and the number of steps you take. But it's difficult to get an accurate read."

In one study, Porcari used a portable metabolic device to get an accurate read on the number of calories burned by 20 volunteers as they walked, ran, did elliptical exercise, and performed basketball drills. He compared that to the numbers from five fitness trackers that the exercisers wore.

The trackers were off by **13 to 60 percent.** "They were okay for walking. They weren't very good for running or on the elliptical, and they were absolutely terrible on the basketball drills. When you get into more complicated movement patterns, the equations really fall apart."

It's best to consider the numbers as relative.

Think of it as similar to the 10,000 steps a day concept. It's not a magic number, but it's a way to know if you seem to generally be moving around less or becoming more sedentary.

There are plenty of numbers you can track more accurately--sets, weight, reps, heart rate.... Calorie burn is one you can skip!

2 WAYS GOALS CAUSE PEOPLE TO STOP EXERCISING

We live in a goal-driven, instant gratification society.

That mindset carries over into exercise, as most people think of exercise as a way to reach a weight loss goal or a performance goal.

"I just ran 3 miles! Maybe I'll run a marathon!"

Some people falter with exercise adherence because unconsciously, they think of it as something they do to lose a certain amount of weight or like the way they look in a swimsuit.

They can get really impatient when they don't reach those goals quickly, not realizing that true fat loss really does take some time.

Weight loss is about calorie balance, rather than about exercising, and that's one reason 80% of people who lose weight gain it back.

For there to be lasting change, there has to be a lasting *habit* change.

Other people quit exercising because they did too much or did it incorrectly and got injured. People are likely to be more competitive in their youth and gravitate toward higher intensity training. (CrossFit, anyone?)

A lot of these exercisers will later have to deal with limits to what their body can tolerate because of the long-term effect of overuse injuries.

They paid a high price in pursuit of their goals.

It's not necessary to beat yourself to a pulp for exercise to deliver its maximum benefits. The leader of the biking group I once belonged to told me, "You should always feel at the end like you could have done more."

Exercise and movement are critical components of a healthy *lifestyle*.

People who exercise consistently do it because they value the fact that it gives them more energy, less pain, the ability to do the things they want to do, keeps them out of the doctor's office, and, yes, it supports weight loss efforts, even if it doesn't burn a lot of calories.

I understand how hard it can be to find time to exercise. The key for me and most people is to schedule it into the week. Decide to reschedule it if you have to, but don't cancel those appointments--make your health and well-being a priority!

Every little bit matters. It doesn't have to be an *hour-long* commitment.

But it is a *life-long* commitment.

My goals? I exercise to be strong, healthy and self-sufficient.

Above all, I work out for the possibility of seeing my 100th birthday.

THE TYRANNY OF 10,000 STEPS

Recently a client told me that she sometimes marches in place beside her bed to get her 10,000 steps before she calls it a night.

DO WE NEED TO GET 10,000 STEPS EVERY DAY?

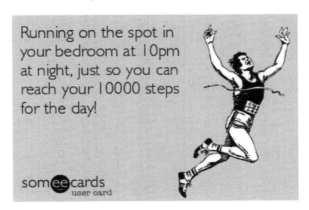

There's actually no science behind that number.

In 1965, a Japanese pedometer company named their product *the "10,000 step meter," apparently choosing that name because the character for "10,000" looks similar to a man walking.*

It's an arbitrary number...a marketing gimmick.

A Harvard researcher studied 16,000 elderly women and found that the ones who walked 4,400 steps per day had much lower premature mortality rates than the ones who were the least active. If they did more, their mortality rates continued to drop, until they reached about 7,500 steps, at which point the rates leveled out.1

But you have to wonder: were the more active women moving more because they felt better and were healthier?

Certainly, walking is good for you--being outside can lift your spirits and the activity can lower blood pressure and improve sleep.

But research is indicating that it's not about the number of steps, it's about the level of movement you get all day.2

Rather than obsessing about steps, the healthier approach is to make sure you don't sit for long periods. My Fitbit reminds me to move if I haven't gotten 250 steps in an hour, something I can rectify simply by going to check the mail or refilling my water bottle.

I use my daily step count as a measure of how active I've been on a given day, compared to most days. Since the pandemic hit, I get fewer than 10,000 steps most days.

A lot of us are working from home more than ever and discovering that we're more sedentary than usual. We have to recognize that this is a particular season of life and deal with it the best we can.

Being fit and healthy shouldn't involve shame for not "meeting certain standards."

That leads to obsessive behavior and frustration with "failing" to meet those standards.

If you *want* to increase your steps, start with adding 500 or so each day. And if that doesn't feel right, do something else good for your body, like yoga or dancing or something you enjoy.

If that includes marching beside your bed....go for it!

Exercise should fit your life, not the other way around.

4 WAYS MULTI-TASKING DOESN'T WORK WITH EXERCISE

I used to pride myself on my multi-tasking ability. It was Katie and Matthew's fault. When you're juggling two babies all by yourself and trying to keep the three of you fed, clothed, *and not crying*, you find yourself desperate for ways to get more done.

Over time, I realized that it actually made me more inefficient. Now we know that when you try to do two things at once, you don't do either as well as if you gave each your full attention.

Exercise is a great example. Trying to do two things at once means you're not getting the best of either.

TRYING TO COMBINE STRENGTH AND ENDURANCE ("CARDIO")

Strength and endurance are two different energy systems--anaerobic and aerobic.

Since strength gains come from 6-12 repetitions, you're not building appreciable muscle strength when you're ramping up the resistance for half an hour on an elliptical machine. Using the arms on the elliptical will help to get your heart rate up, but your arms won't get stronger, and the distraction of moving your arms back and forth is likely to distract your body from using your lower body more.

I know your spin instructor is telling you to crank up the resistance on that bike but **resist**! (*see what I did there?*) There's way too much stress on your knees when you ramp up the resistance on a bike. Knees aren't designed to tolerate that shear force-- ask any cyclist.

It's like when people tried to add weights to step classes. No muscle got built while people were flinging weights around as they stepped up and down...but some joints got stressed out!

People who only walk or run for exercise are surprised to discover that their legs aren't very strong. Their legs might have a lot of endurance but little strength. That's because they're using their *aerobic* system and not *anaerobic*--there's no progressive load.

Better to do workouts geared for either strength or endurance. You'll get more results quicker--with less risk of injury!

TRYING TO COMBINE STRENGTH AND BALANCE

There's a definite place for balance training, especially when it comes to strengthening stabilizers. But the weight I press overhead is going to be a lot less if I'm only standing on one foot. **There's a trade-off between strength and stability.** So consider the goal--if you want to do a stronger press, do it on two feet. If you want to challenge stability, do it on one.

And if you want to do anything on a BOSU, all I can say is "WHY????"

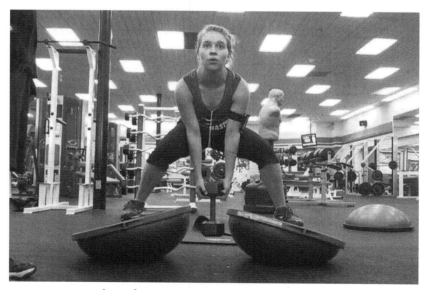

unless, of course, your goal is better BOSUing....

TRYING TO COMBINE STRENGTH AND POWER

This happens all the time with medicine balls but it can be any exercise with a power component. The rule of thumb is that a medicine ball should weigh 10% of your body weight. You can't generate power well if you're wrangling with the weight.

Imagine how much farther you could throw a 1# ball than a 5# ball. Power training is all about creating an explosive movement.

TRYING TO COMBINE DISTRACTIONS WITH... ANY EXERCISE

I'll never forget the new client who asked me, as she surveyed a room full of cardio machines, "Which one of these can I do and knit at the same time?"

If you're doing cardio at the right level, you *should* be moving too much to read... or knit. Listening to music is good because you're not expecting to remember any of it. Listening to a podcast is trickier because you're unlikely to remember details, depending on the type and intensity of the exercise.

Distracted exercise can be dangerous. More people are injured while talking on the phone and walking than while driving. When you're distracted, you're no longer paying attention to your form or posture.

Trying to do two things at one time leads to doing both poorly—or at least really poorly at one.

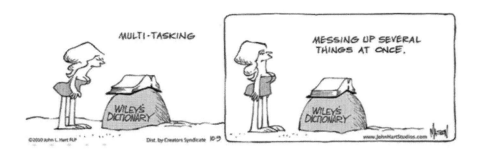

NO, YOU CAN'T CREATE "LONG, LEAN MUSCLES"

I thought everyone by now knew that you can't make your muscles "long"--your mom and dad got to decide that one. Some people have relatively longer muscle-to-tendon ratios but *that's something you can't change.*

And muscle is.... well, muscle. It's lean by definition. There can be some fat marbling in there but that's...well, fat. You can't have fat muscle or lean muscle, it's **muscle**.

But I'm still seeing ads like this:

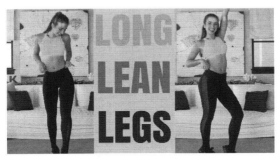

Longer legs? Sign me up!

The "long, lean muscle" terminology developed when women were afraid that strength training would build a lot of muscle and make them "bulky."

A **lot** of work goes into building an appreciable amount of muscle. It means a high volume of sets in daily strength training, a protocol most people don't use.

Furthermore, women don't have the testosterone needed to build a lot of muscle--neither do a lot of men!

Strength training, using compound movements, like squats, lunges, pulls and pushes, is not only critical to good health and function, it's your friend when you're trying to lose fat and gain muscle. It helps preserve muscle so that you don't lose fat and muscle at the same time.

Training for muscle strength and training for muscle size are completely different protocols. If the training plan fits the goal, there's no reason to fear strength training.

Generally, the "bulky" look comes from the layer of *fat* that's over the muscle—reducing the fat isn't easy, either. Your efforts are affected by stress, sleep, nutrition quality, hormones, genetics, and your general health.

The one part you absolutely can not control is the length of your muscles...or your legs!

TOO OLD FOR "THE FRESHMAN 15"?
HOW ABOUT "THE FROSTY 15"?

I used to try to get my dad to work out and he'd smile at me tolerantly and say, "I work in the yard and stay strong hauling stuff like bags of fertilizer...."

I'd try to convince him that he was getting weaker each winter and each spring would be harder.

Well, you know what they say about the cobbler's children....

Researchers at the University of Liverpool wanted to see how we're affected by inactivity--the sort we experience over the holidays or during periods of winter or weather unfavorable to exercise.

The Results:

- Both the younger and older groups studied lost leg strength, gained body fat, and lost muscle size and bone mass.
- Since the older group generally had more body fat and less muscle to start with, their health was more affected.
- Cardiorespiratory fitness of the older group declined twice as much as the younger group.

The Good News:

As long as you can get to some weights, you can maintain your strength, rain or shine, all year long. Strength training alone can help mitigate cardiovascular fitness losses.

You still need to keep moving, too. Make sure you don't sit still for more than 30 minutes at a time. Make multiple trips up and down stairs. Put on some music and dance. Get a kettlebell and do a workout--there's so much you can do with a kettlebell!

It's important to your health to not lose fitness over the winter--in addition to staying fit, exercising and staying active will strengthen your immune system and keep good habits going.

Then, in a few weeks, you'll be ready to Spring into action!

THE CROSSOVER EFFECT
THE KEY TO WORKING AROUND
AN INJURY

Have you ever had an injury that threatened to keep you out of action?

Good news--continuing to work out can help keep that injured body part strong.

The "Crossover Effect" is neurological and it refers to the way that training, say your healthy left leg, will help keep your injured right leg strong. It's been reported in a host of studies, dating back to 1894.1

> "...the degree of strength gained in the untrained limb is usually proportional to that gained in the trained limb. Training variations such as speed, intensity, and contraction type contribute to the wide range of strength transfer reported, though a 2006 meta-analysis found that **the average reported strength gain in the untrained limb was 7.6%, ... roughly a third of the gains in the trained limb.**"

We've had clients come in wearing walking casts, shoulder slings, knee braces, and boots. They recover faster because they keep moving and keep their uninjured body parts strong. And it keeps up their total body conditioning.2

> "When you work one side of the body, there is a 30-40% neurological crossover on the opposite side. By strengthening the right shoulder, you're also strengthening the left side, even if you don't move it at all. The same principle also applies to muscle activation and range of motion. If you're feeling stuck or you're suffering from an injury, try working the opposite limb or side of the body. If it's safe to do

so, you can also try your activity or your sport with your non-dominant hand. Not only does it keep you in the game, but it also helps strengthen the opposing area without any risk of injury."

The next time you're dealing with an injury, don't let it get you down. Not only can you keep going, you *should*!

EXERCISE, DEPRESSION, AND
THE DIFFERENCE A COACH MAKES

Recently I asked a client how he was feeling, having come in a few weeks before with shoulder pain, postural issues, and knee pain.

He paused, looked me in the eye and said, "This is going to sound strange but my mood is better."

It's been recognized for some time that exercise is an effective treatment for depression. One theory is that it improves posture and a less depressed posture leads to feeling less depressed.

Or is it a biochemical reaction--the "runner's high" that some experience post-workout from an increased level of endocannabinoids, sometimes referred to as "endorphins"?

Jacob Meyer, an assistant professor of kinesiology at Iowa State University in Ames, began a study of endocannabinoids and the runner's high.1

"Multiple studies show that **physically active people are more apt to report being happy than sedentary people and are less likely to experience anxiety or depression....regular exercise reduced the symptoms of depression as effectively as antidepressant medications....** Created in many of our body's tissues all the time, endocannabinoids bind to specialized receptors in our brains and nervous systems and help to increase calm and improve moods....People with diagnoses of depression often have relatively low levels of endocannabinoids in their blood... while mice and rats born with malfunctioning endocannabinoid receptors typically develop a kind of rodent depression."

He set up a study in which women with major depression did workouts on a stationary bike. The workout intensity varied from easy to draining. Most of the time, they were coached as to which level of intensity to work. Other times, they could work at any intensity they chose.

> "After both workouts, the women reported feeling less depressed and worried. But only when they had followed instructions to pedal moderately did their blood show increases in endocannabinoids. When they had exercised at their preferred pace, even if it was moderate, endocannabinoid levels remained unchanged. What these results suggest, Dr. Meyer says, is that **being coached and supervised leads to different impacts on our bodies and minds than working at our own pace, whatever that pace might be**...Why the prescribed exercise should have increased endocannabinoids, though, while the go-as-you-please workout did not is still mysterious...It may be that our brains recognize when a workout's intensity is not one we would voluntarily choose and prompt the release of substances that make the effort more tolerable.

> ...any exercise is better for mental health than none. **'It might be helpful for people suffering from depression to work with a personal trainer or other fitness professional' who can supervise the sessions,'** he says."

There is power in human connection. But having a coach is different from having a workout buddy.

A coach understands your goals and struggles and provides a sturdy support system, often believing in you when you don't believe in yourself. (Dozens of times clients have said, "I would NEVER have done that on my own!") Life really does begin outside your comfort zone.

Having a coach takes you to the next level. I have a business coach who pushes me to do things that make me squirm and whose expertise I trust. I consider it an *investment*, not an expense.

If you've never had a coach, it's time to give it a try!

ARE YOU OUT OF BALANCE?
HERE'S HOW TO FIX IT

A lot of our lives is spent on one leg—walking, running, going up stairs, stepping up onto a curb....

That's why we do a lot of training on one leg. The ability to move and stabilize well on one leg is so important that evaluating it is part of our assessment process.

Most people struggle with it. Some are surprised by the challenge, saying, "Wow, my balance isn't good." Their reaction is interesting--it's as if they're either thinking, "I'm old and losing my balance." or "There's something wrong with me." They think balance is a quality they've lost, like losing their eyesight--something they have no control over.

There are lots of reasons to have trouble with balance but overwhelmingly the one we most often see is an issue of muscle balance--inadequate strength in certain muscles.

When muscles are weak or inhibited, there's a lack of muscle balance around joints that throws you off balance. Often, it's an issue of weakness in the muscles on the sides of the hips, weak glutes, and tight hip flexors.

This is what we typically see--alignment and weakness of the hip causes the leg to turn in, collapsing the arch and causing the foot to turn out. That can lead to plantar fasciitis. And hip and knee pain. And sciatic pain.

That's where bunions come from, by the way. We do an InBody scan first thing with all new clients. If I look down at someone's bare feet and see bunions, I know I'll be seeing hip issues later in the assessment.

The solution?

The first thing to address is the hip weakness. We do that with a variety of exercises, including hinges, squats, lunges, side planks, and step ups.

Once the hips are stronger, the feet don't have so much pressure on them. The arch can get stronger and lift back up again. We work on the posterior tibialis (along the shin) and strengthening the big toe.

Most people don't really use their toes anymore, *especially if they turn their feet out when they walk.* But the big toe is critical for balance.

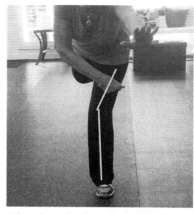

This client had really bad knee and hip pain.

Try it! Stand up and pick up one foot. Can you feel the difference it makes to press your big toe into the ground?

Balance also improves with work on posture and walking mechanics.

Actually, **balance simply gets better by virtue of getting stronger--all over.** You'll also discover that **when you are working to improve your balance, lots of other things get better, too--like achy joints and muscles.**

So you can add balance to the long list of things that a well-balanced strength training program improves.... pun somewhat intended....

COULD YOU FORGET ABOUT "EXERCISE" AND JUST DO THIS?

It doesn't have to be "exercise." Simply moving can make you happier.

Kelly McGonigal says in her book, The Joy Of Movement,1

> "Around the world, people who are physically active are happier and more satisfied with their lives.... whether their preferred activity is walking, running, swimming, dancing, biking, playing sports, lifting weights, or practicing yoga. People who are regularly active have a stronger sense of purpose, and they experience more gratitude, love, and hope. They feel more connected to their communities, are less likely to suffer from loneliness or become depressed. These benefits are seen throughout the lifespan. They apply to every socioeconomic strata and appear to be culturally universal... They have been demonstrated in people with chronic pain, physical disabilities, serious mental and physical illnesses, and even among patients in hospice care. The joys described above—from hope and meaning to belonging— are *linked... to movement, not to fitness.*"

"HOPE MOLECULES"

It's not about endorphins.

> "Physical activity influences many other brain chemicals, including those that give you energy, alleviate worry, and help you bond with others. It reduces inflammation in the brain, which over time can protect against depression, anxiety, and loneliness. Regular exercise

also remodels the physical structure of your brain to make you more receptive to joy and social connection. These neurological changes rival those observed in the most cutting-edge treatments for both depression and addiction. The mind-altering effects of exercise are even embedded in your musculature. During physical activity, muscles secrete hormones into your bloodstream that make your brain more resilient to stress. Scientists call them 'hope molecules.'"

movement will give you access to joy that will dramatically improve the quality of your life help support mental health and create more meaning and belonging

KELLY MCGONIGAL, PHD

Why are so many people resistant? All you gotta do is move. McGonigal says:

"Anything that keeps you moving and increases your heart rate is enough to trigger nature's reward for not giving up. There's no objective measure of performance you must achieve, no pace or distance you need to reach, that determines whether you experience an exercise-induced euphoria. **You just have to do something that is moderately difficult for you and stick with it for at least twenty minutes. That's because the runner's high isn't a running high. It's a persistence high.**"

Sociologist Emile Durkheim described the bonding that people feel from moving together as "collective effervescence."

McGonigal says it's

> "...why fitness friendships and sports teams feel like family; why social movements that include physical movement inspire greater solidarity and hope; and why individuals feel empowered when they join others to walk, run, or ride for a cure."

Movement is part of the human experience.

> "We overcome obstacles, break through barriers, and walk through fire. We carry burdens, reach out for help, and lift one another up. This is how we humans talk about bravery and resilience. When we are faced with adversity or doubting our own strength, it can help to feel these actions in our bodies. Sometimes we need to climb an actual hill, pull ourselves up, or work together to shoulder a heavy load to know that these traits are part of us."

Walk, dance, run, skip...simply revel in the joy of movement!

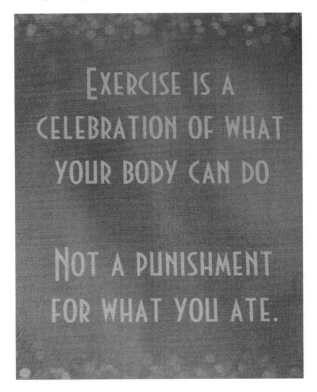

NUTRITION

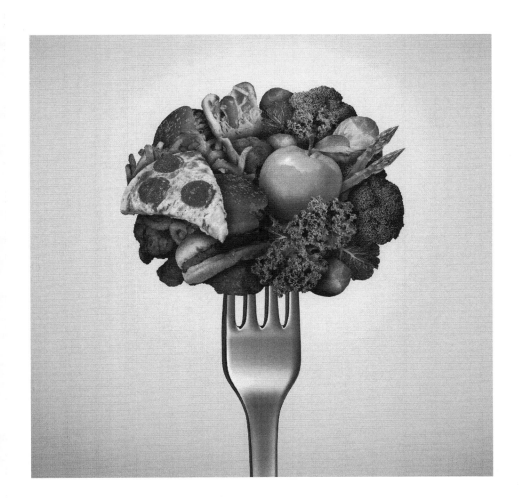

SIMPLY IRRESISTIBLE.....

If you've ever felt like you have no self-control around certain foods, you'll be interested to know that there's a reason for that, and it's not that you just don't have any will-power.

Food manufacturers have perfected the art of making their foods irresistible. Yep, we're being manipulated by the food industry and blissfully unaware.

The rise of ultra-processed foods has coincided with growing rates of obesity, leading many to suspect that they've played a big role in our growing waistlines.

But is it something about the highly processed nature of these foods itself that drives people to overeat? A new study suggests the answer is YES. 1.

> "The study...is the first randomized, controlled trial to show that eating a diet made up of ultra-processed foods actually drives people to overeat and gain weight compared with a diet made up of whole or minimally processed foods.
>
> Study participants on the ultra-processed diet ate an average of 508 calories more per day and ended up gaining an average of 2 pounds over a two-week period. People on the unprocessed diet, meanwhile, ended up losing about 2 pounds on average over a two-week period......
>
> 'The difference in weight gain for one [group] and weight loss for the other during these two periods is phenomenal. We haven't seen anything like this.'"

What *are* "processed foods"?

"...ultra-processed foods include more than just the obvious suspects, like chips, candy, packaged desserts and ready-to-eat meals..... foods that some consumers might find surprising, including Honey Nut Cheerios and other breakfast cereals, packaged white bread, jarred sauces, yogurt with added fruit, and frozen sausages and other reconstituted meat products."

Participants eating unprocessed foods had higher levels of an appetite suppressing hormone and lower levels of a hunger hormone.

The reverse was true of those who ate processed food. People ate much faster on the processed food diet, possibly because the food was softer and easier to chew. It was easy to consume a lot before their brain got the message that they'd had enough to eat!

If you want to learn more about how the food industry is manipulating us, check out these videos:

Why We Can't Stop Eating Unhealthy Foods

https://www.youtube.com/watch?v=wTNlHyjip94&feature=youtu.be

The Science of Addictive Food

https://www.youtube.com/watch?v=4cpdb78pWl4&feature=youtu.be

Food Addiction: Is The Food Industry Creating An Epidemic?

https://www.youtube.com/watch?v=uMbAwahgm0E&feature=youtu.be

INSTEAD OF AN ANTIOXIDANT
TAKE A PLACEBO?

We hear a lot of talk about antioxidants, but when it comes to strength training, antioxidant supplements may be working against you.1

> "....free radicals and the resulting oxidation is normal to some degree, but when there's an overload...it leads to chronic and degenerative illnesses, including cancer, rheumatoid arthritis, and autoimmune disorders.

> You also age faster...Enter antioxidants. Your body already produces a bunch, but it surely helps to stimulate that process in other ways, particularly by staying active, eating your veggies, getting enough sleep, implementing de-stress tactics, and supplementing with antioxidant vitamins like C and E.

> However, a new study reveals, if you're looking to increase muscle mass, you may want to leave that last item off your antioxidant to-do list....**only the placebo group—those weight lifting but not taking any antioxidant supplements—saw an increase in muscle mass and a loss in fat. They boosted their lean muscle by just over three pounds while losing about 1.5 pounds of fat....the people taking the antioxidant supplements did not experience any significant increase in muscle or decrease in fat....**

> When you lift weights, you produce oxidative stress, too. But that's not a bad thing, because it helps your muscles use protein better...So, if you decrease your oxidative stress too much—by taking those vitamins, for example—then you can't use protein as effectively.... to increase muscle mass efficiently, you need to utilize protein for muscle building and recovery....

So **even if you're consuming the correct amount of protein for your strength efforts, but if you're taking antioxidants, that protein won't translate into muscle mass gains**.....if you're a healthy young person and want to improve body composition by lifting weights, you should avoid supplementation of antioxidants like vitamin C and E…"

If your life feels empty without pills, *there's still one that seems to have no side effects*-the placebo. *Time* magazine reports, 2

"Nearly twice as many people in the trial who **knowingly received placebo pills reported experiencing adequate symptom relief,** compared to the people who received no treatment.... **the men and women taking the placebo also doubled their rates of improvement to a point that was about equal to the effects of two IBS medications**...

…entrepreneurs are beginning to pay attention, and you can now buy placebo pills on Amazon for $8 to $15 a bottle.....the **effect appears to be stronger if people are told a medication is hard to get or expensive, and color may also matter, with people responding better to blue pills as sedatives and white pills for pain**....

Jeni Danto, a therapist and mother of five children ages 11 to 17, created a parenting hack called Magic Feel Good, which you can buy on Amazon for $8.99. When her children were younger, it seemed that every week one child or another was suffering from phantom pain or a suspicious tummy ache before school. If she and her husband Akiva determined that the complaints weren't serious or even real, Akiva would slip into the kitchen and stir up a mixture of orange juice, grape juice and honey and then bring it to their child in a medicine cup, calling it 'Magic Feel Good.'...

'Placebo is not magic,' says Alia Crum, principal investigator at the Stanford Mind & Body Lab... '**We view placebo effect as the product of your body's ability to heal, which is activated by our mind-sets and expectations to heal, and shaped by medical ritual, branding of drugs and the words doctors say.'**"

You have to love a medicine whose only side effect is that you feel better!

3 NUTRITION SOURCES YOU CAN TRUST

Keto, paleo, high carb, high fat, fasting, Whole30, eat for your blood type....

There's so much noise in the nutrition space that one of my friends exclaimed, "You never know what to believe--it's always changing!"

Actually, that's not true. Basic nutrition principles have remained the same for a long time. Calories count. Eat unprocessed food. Focus on vegetables.

But people are looking for a magic formula that will let them eat as much as they want of whatever they want OR make the weight they want to lose fall off of them in record time.

And there are LOTS of people ready to take advantage of that magical thinking with their diets and eating protocols.

There are 3 sources you can trust, where you can get questions on any aspect of nutrition answered.

PRECISION NUTRITION

John Berardi does an amazing job of distilling the pros and cons of all kinds of nutrition subjects, without advocating any agenda. The website is geared to training nutrition coaches but their article archive is thorough and well researched. 1

You'll find subjects like, "Can Eating Too Little Actually Damage Your Metabolism?" and "Should You Quit Drinking Diet Soda?"

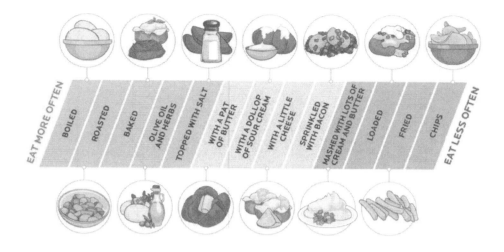

CENTER FOR SCIENCE IN THE PUBLIC INTEREST

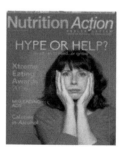

CSPI is like the *Consumer Reports* of nutrition. They publish the Nutrition Action newsletter and are on the lookout for shady practices that consumers need to be aware of when it comes to the food they buy in stores and restaurants.

Sign up for their weekly newsletter or their monthly, *Nutrition Action Health Letter.2* The articles are entertaining and make learning about health and nutrition fun--like "Xtreme Eating: America's Worst Restaurant Meals," "Big Fat Myths," and "Servings on Steroids."

HOW TO EAT: ALL YOUR FOOD AND DIET QUESTIONS ANSWERED

The excerpts I have read from this book have been phenomenal. 3

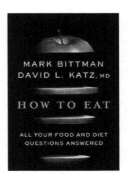

"Is there a "diet" that leaves all the others in the dust? It would be truer to say that **we know eating patterns that beat out other diets — but as soon as we move in that sensible, defensible direction, all the pixie dust drops out of the equation; it doesn't sound like magic. Sadly, most people are convinced they want pixie dust, no matter how many times false promises about its magical powers have let them down, and no matter how simple good eating is shown to be. Whenever we're comparing contemporary diets, from intermittent fasting to Whole30, there are commercial interests attached. But the simple truth is that all "good" diets share the same principles: They focus on foods that are close to nature, minimally processed, and plant predominant — what we call a whole-food, plant-predominant diet."**

They took the words right out of my mouth!

There are lots of good resources out there, but if you're looking for nutrition answers, these are great places to start and sources you can trust.

THIS KIND OF CARB CAN HELP YOU LOSE WEIGHT

Have you ever heard of resistant starch?

It's a type of carbohydrate that passes through the small intestine without being digested. Studies suggest that it can boost immunity, improve blood sugar control, and lower cancer risk. Body fat was reduced by up to 45% in an animal study, as reported in *Critical Reviews in Food Science and Nutrition*.

There's a lot to gain...and maybe lose...by finding a way to incorporate more resistant starch in your diet--especially since it also improves gut flora and helps with feeling full.

Here are some sources:

- **Raw oats**—I use raw oats in muesli, snack bites, and overnight oats.

- **White beans**--Cannellini beans are my favorite. You can throw them into salads and soups. They're also good as a stand-alone side dish. They're delicious cooked with garlic and rosemary.

- **Lentils**--Lentils are versatile and a half cup has 9 grams of protein.

- **Underripe bananas**--The carbohydrate in bananas converts from starch to sugar as the banana turns from green to yellow. That also means that green bananas aren't very palatable, in my humble opinion. Corn, on the other hand, owes its "just picked" sweetness to a high percentage of sugar. But the longer it sits after harvesting, the more its sugar converts to starch.

- **Cold pasta and potatoes**--I routinely cook these two ahead of time so I can refrigerate them overnight. Once cooled, their starch becomes resistant starch. One study found a 57% increase in resistant starch after refrigerating potatoes overnight. The amount of resistant starch increases as the length of refrigeration increases. This trick also works for rice.

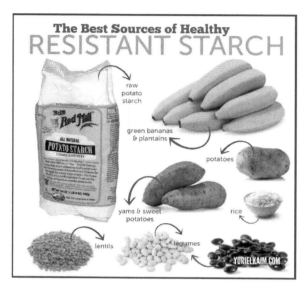

Little things add up to big things—ever read The Compound Effect about the difference 1% can make?

When there are substitutions and prep tweaks that can make a difference, why not give it a whirl?

3 THINGS THAT WILL IMPROVE YOUR IMMUNITY--WITHOUT SUPPLEMENTS

You may have heard of supplements that claim to "improve immunity." In the absence of nutritional deficiencies, it's a waste of money and could be harmful if they create nutritional imbalances or overdoses.

How about improving your resilience and immunity safely and effectively?

Practice Positivity--It Worked For the Nuns The University of Kentucky studied entry statements of nuns who were about 22 years old at the time. *By the age of 85, 97% of the nuns whose entries contained the most positive content were still alive, vs 52% of the least positive. By age 93, 52% of the positive entrants were still alive vs 18% of the least cheerful.* Similarly, a study of 96 famous psychologists found that those who used more positive words lived on average 6 years longer than those who used more negative words.

Eat Real Food In 1700, sugar consumption per person was 5 pounds per person per *year*. Today the average American consumes 3 pounds per *week*.

Not only does sugar take the place of nutritious food, it's linked to increasing depression. Our consumption of *processed foods* is responsible for increasing rates of obesity, high blood pressure and diabetes.

Exercise! Being physically active is like a wonder drug. Kate Hefferon says in Positive Psychology and the Body, exercise can

> "....produce positive emotions, self-efficacy, mastery and overall flourishing. In terms of reducing, activity has been found to **lower**

the risk of developing obesity, cardiovascular disease, coronary heart disease, stroke, diabetes (type 2), osteoporosis, certain sleep disorders, high blood pressure (e.g. blood pressure reduces for up to 12 hours post exercise), certain cancers (colon, breast, rectal, lung, prostate, endometrial) and even premature death.

Exercise can also be used to **enhance immune system functioning**, however, there appears to be a J-shape relationship, such that moderate, *chronic levels of activity are better in the promotion of immune system functioning than chronic, high intensity.*

In terms of *producing*, physical activity has been linked to...wellbeing including: positive emotions, self-esteem, body image, cognitive functioning, psychological wellbeing, posttraumatic growth, flow, purpose in life and many, many more concepts."

Good health is easy to take for granted until you don't have it.

We should treat it like the treasure it is.

WEIGHT
LOSS

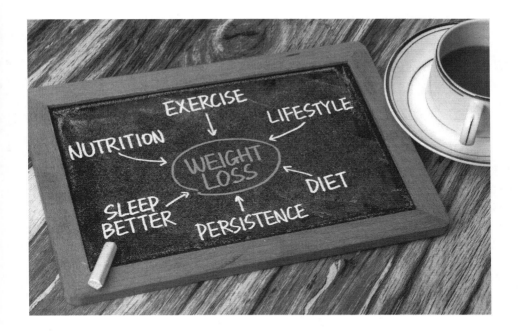

WHY I DON'T BELIEVE IN
WEIGHT LOSS CHALLENGES

When you think about losing weight, what comes to mind? Being hungry? Eating special meals? Not being allowed to have foods you love? Have you ever heard someone say "Woo hoo! I'm going on a diet!"?

The idea is that once you've spent a certain amount of time being deprived of the foods you love, you'll reach a goal weight.

And then....you'll love your life? Your body? You'll be happy? Why do 85% of people gain back the weight they lost?

Josh Hillis writes on health, nutrition and weight loss. He suggests that we focus on the process, rather than the goal. What he says here applies beautifully to weight loss.1

> "Most of us approach goals like we'll only be the kind of person we want to be" after we hit the goal.
>
> In reality, we get to be the kind of person we want to be every time we take actions in line with that value. Every workout, we're being strength. Every milestone. Not just the last one.

> There is no ending to becoming the kind of person we want to be. It's not a goal, it's a daily practice.

> The irony is that *people tend to get better results when they're focused on process based goals (like doing the work) instead of outcome goals (like looking a certain way).*

Paradoxically, people who over-value the end result often get disheartened and quit, when they don't hit their goals fast enough, or maybe miss a milestone on the way to their goals. They get thrown by each and every (normal) bump in the road.

On the flip-side, people get awesome results when they simply focus on doing the work. When people just focus on doing the work:

- They do more work
- They do higher quality work
- They do more consistent work

If you just focus on doing the work in the gym every day, you'll get stronger.

Also, you might find it to be more empowering, more fun, and have a drastically more positive impact on your relationship to your body. Instead of being entirely focused on some idealized body standard, your gym work can **simply be an expression of being the kind of person you want to be.**"

When it comes to weight loss, lasting change comes from making lasting changes.

There's a sort of "finish line" mentality about reaching a goal weight. But crossing that line isn't really a finish line. That's why losing weight is said to be easier than keeping it off.

I'm sure you've seen promises out there to "Lose 12 Pounds In 6 Weeks" or contests where gyms and workplaces hand out prizes for the people who lose the most weight in a given time--who cross that finish line first. There's no magic diet and certainly no magic exercise plan that will create quick and lasting weight loss. The Biggest Losers are examples of people whose extreme exercise and diet plans--trying to lose the most the fastest--resulted in people who are now back where they started.

Practicing new habits gives us the opportunity to celebrate success daily--eating a more nutritious breakfast, getting more sleep, learning what "hungry" and "enough" feel like, discovering new vegetables and ways to cook, managing stress without using food.... These are the habits that lead to long term weight loss.

And it teaches us patience.

"THE ROAD LESS STUPID" TO WEIGHT LOSS

I recently discovered the Story Brand website and podcast. If you are involved in business, you will LOVE this podcast. It's the only one I listen to that I regularly pause to make notes.

This one caught my attention because of the comparisons between business strategies and weight loss strategies.

Keith Cunningham is a brilliant business guru and the interview was related to his book, The Road Less Stupid.

Episode 159 Keith Cunningham—5 Simple Ideas That Will Help You Avoid Dumb Business Mistakes

At the 36 minute mark, quoting:

> "The hardest work I do is figuring out what in the world is the problem that I've got. If you keep drilling deep enough you'll find the core, root problem and the reason people go on diets and it doesn't work is because they're *tactical* in their solutions.... 'I want to lose 20 pounds.' The first thing they do is think, 'What do I need to do?' Their brain goes to 'I need to join a gym....I need to get an elliptical trainer for my house....I need a Peloton...if I just had a trainer...if I just had Oprah's newest diet book, then I could lose....'
>
> **Every one of those is tactical and the reason they're not successful in losing the weight is because they haven't identified the core, root problem. Instead they're solving for the symptom, so they're building a machine for the problem that isn't.**

If the symptom is 'I'm 20 pounds overweight.' maybe the question becomes

'Why isn't this already solved?'

'How did this become a symptom to begin with?'

'What are the obstacles or constraints that are preventing me from weighing less?'

'If I could only _____ I could solve this problem.'

'If I only had _____ I could solve this problem.'

'Whose support do I need?"

'What assumptions am I making?'

All of these questions are designed to help you get clarity on what the problem is......

What I'm looking for is clarity on 'what are the things that are preventing me from actually losing the weight....'"

So if you've decided to make changes to become healthier, whether it's losing weight, sleeping more, getting stronger and more fit, reducing stress, making better food choices....doesn't it make SO much sense to start with

"What got me here?"

"What has kept me here?"

Weight loss is a journey. The first step is evaluating where you're starting.

Successfully reaching the destination requires a well-prepared roadmap.

DOES EXERCISE AFFECT WEIGHT LOSS?

The idea that weight loss is the goal of exercise is a myth that just won't go away--mostly because the fitness industry perpetuates it. It's been an effective way to sell gym memberships. *Nutrition Action*1 reports,

> "*Following the workout, as your body recovers, your metabolism stays elevated so you're continuing to burn more calories and more fat hours after the workout is over," says the video at* OrangetheoryFitness.com, *an exercise program designed to boost 'afterburn'.*

Exercising at a high intensity or for a prolonged period of time at a moderate intensity can increase afterburn,'" says Jenna Gillen, assistant professor of kinesiology and physical education at the University of Toronto. 'But intensity has the most impact.'

Still, **that impact is modest**...when men exercised for 80 minutes, afterburn was roughly twice as high when they switched from a lower to a higher intensity. But afterburn accounted for **only about 6 percent of the total calories** burned during and after the hardest workout.

'You'll hear claims that you burn 40 to 50 percent more calories than you would at rest due to afterburn, but the effect is much more subtle.'

Afterburn does help explain why you can save time if you work out at a higher intensity. Gillen's team had men either cycle at moderate intensity for 50 minutes or do 20 minutes of high-intensity interval cycling... 'They didn't burn as many calories during the high-intensity interval training as when they did the longer, moderate-intensity exercise,' says Gillen.

But their **afterburn was about 100 calories higher after the high-intensity intervals. 'So, over a 24-hour period, calorie burning was similar.'** Bottom Line: Afterburn is real, but its contribution to total calorie burn is overstated.

People start exercising, expecting the weight to fall off of them as a result, and then get frustrated and quit because "it didn't work."

You can't outrun your fork

Again, from *Nutrition Action,*

> "To find out why, researchers randomly assigned 171 sedentary people with overweight or obesity to burn:
>
> A: no extra calories
>
> B: roughly 100 extra calories a day, or
>
> C: roughly 250 extra calories a day.
>
> After six months, group A had lost 1/2 pound, group B had lost about 1 pound, and group C had lost 3 1/2 pounds.
>
> Based on how much the groups exercised, the researchers calculated that group B should have lost another 3 pounds and group C should have lost another 6 pounds....
>
> The people in groups B and C 'compensated' for the exercise by eating roughly 100 extra calories a day....

If you want to lose weight, eat less.

Exercise to lower your risk of type 2 diabetes, heart disease, stroke, some cancers, bone loss, muscle loss, and more."

5 REASONS COUNTING CALORIES IS OBSOLETE

More than two-thirds of American adults are overweight or obese and we live in a state that is tied with Arkansas and Mississippi for being the second fattest state in the country. (Oklahoma is #1) A third of this population is trying to lose weight by "dieting" and "counting calories."

The Mosaic Science Podcast describes why calorie counting is so inaccurate.1

- There's a difference between the number of calories in a food and the number your body will extract. Calorie counts don't make that distinction.

- Cooking affects how many calories your body will absorb. Preferring your steak well done, as opposed to rare, means the same size portion has more calories. Also, cooking rice and then refrigerating it overnight can more than halve the available calories.

- Processing food makes calories more available to your body by breaking down the cell walls of the food. For instance, eating raw peanuts results in fewer *available* calories than an equivalent amount of processed peanut butter.

- It's really hard to know how many calories your body needs at a base level. Factors like height, body fat, hormone levels, stress, prescription drugs, liver size, and sleep can dramatically affect your calorie requirements.

- Researchers used twin studies and discovered that gut microbes can make the difference in who gains weight and who doesn't, even when eating exactly the same diet.

    "Take the case of the woman who gained more than 40 lbs after receiving a transplant of gut microbes from her overweight teenage daughter. The transplant successfully treated the mother's intestinal infection of *Clostridium difficile*, which had resisted antibiotics.

But, as of the study's publication last year, she hadn't been able to shed the excess weight through diet or exercise. The only aspect of her physiology that had changed was her gut microbes."2

Calorie counts are a quick way to compare one food to another. I hastily put back a wrap sandwich at Trader Joe's when I read it had over 700 calories!

And tracking what you eat can discourage overeating because it makes you eat ***consciously***. (Hmmm....do I want to add another Oreo to this total....?)

Having lost 10 pounds last year, I learned the most effective approach **for me** was

- reducing portion size
- increasing the number of home cooked meals and *focusing on vegetables*
- avoiding processed foods
- reducing alcohol consumption

The hardest thing of all? Being patient. It. Was. Slow. Sometimes I was so frustrated. But I kept trusting the process and it works.

It takes time to make the new practices habits, but once you do, you have a healthier lifestyle that won't ever have to deal with counting calories.

ANY DIET WORKS…
AS LONG AS IT DOESN'T INCLUDE
THIS ONE THING

It's been said that you can lose weight on any diet--even "The Brownie Diet"-- because simply being on a diet makes you more conscious of what you eat and restricts your choices.

Low-carb, high fat, keto, paleo, high-protein, low-fat, plant-based, vegan...the issue isn't whether you'll lose weight, **the issue is about whether you can eat that way for a lifetime.**

The one thing that all of those diets have in common is restriction of **ultra-processed foods.**

A recent study by Kevin Hall and colleagues supports that point in the most rigorous way possible. They locked volunteers inside a metabolic ward for four weeks and accounted for every bite of food. Here's how the *New York Times Magazine* describes the experiment:1

> "They were each randomly assigned to one of two groups. One ate meals consisting primarily of **ultra-processed foods, including many that people typically consider healthy: Honey Nut Cheerios, Yoplait yogurt, and precooked frozen eggs.**
>
> The other group ate mostly unprocessed foods, including oatmeal, roast beef, Greek yogurt, fresh scrambled eggs, and barley. The meals offered to each group contained an equivalent number of calories and proportions of carbohydrates, fat, and sugar; participants ate as much as they wanted. After two weeks, the groups switched diets.

On the ultra-processed diet, the subjects on average consumed 500 more calories a day and gained two pounds."

Processed food currently accounts for 57% of the American diet.

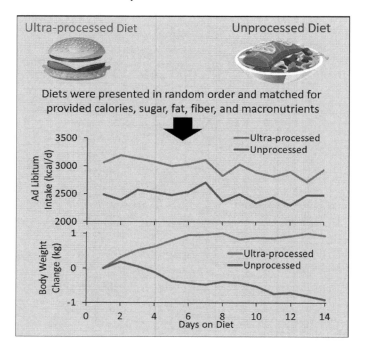

The researchers concluded

> "...our data suggest that **eliminating ultra-processed foods from the diet decreases energy intake and results in weight loss, whereas a diet with a large proportion of ultra-processed food increases energy intake and leads to weight gain.** ...limiting consumption of ultra-processed foods may be an effective strategy for obesity prevention and treatment. Such a recommendation could potentially be embraced across a wide variety of healthy dietary approaches including low- carb, low-fat, plant-based, or animal-based diets."

The researchers didn't address why processed foods lead to weight gain but a couple of theories have been advanced by others. **One is that processed foods are designed to have a combination of fat and salt that make you want to keep eating...** *"Betcha can't eat just one!"*

Another factor is that processed foods are easily digested--the processing essentially "pre-digests" them to a point--so that **the human body doesn't need to spend as much energy for digestion**.

The Thermic Effect Of Food (TEF) is one of the greatest sources of calorie expenditure for the human body.

Imagine being hungry and your options are to have Cheez-Its crackers, which are mostly white flour, sugars, salt and artificial flavors, or a piece of whole grain bread with peanut butter that is simply ground peanuts. Even if the caloric count for a serving is the same, the crackers would more likely predispose you to overeat and because they're so processed, you'd spend fewer calories digesting them. So, the crackers "cost" you more if you're trying to reduce calories.

It's smart to avoid ultra-processed food—the sort of packaged fare containing artificial flavorings and ingredients you wouldn't find in your kitchen—that makes processed food cheap, convenient, tasty, shelf-stable — and popular.

Once you commit to ridding your diet of ultra-processed food, you're likely to discover plenty of ways to create options that are better choices, equally convenient, and not so irresistible.

3 MYTHS ABOUT WEIGHT LOSS & METABOLISM

Once upon a time, we advised people who wanted to lose weight to eat 5 smaller meals a day instead of the usual 3. The belief was that each feeding "stoked the metabolic fire" and that there would be a general increase in metabolism, and hence, calorie burn.

*It turns out.....*the calories spent in digestion are roughly the same, whether they are consumed in 3 meals or 5 smaller meals. It's very easy for those smaller meals to be not-so-small (and the calorie intake higher). Research showed ***people who ate 3 meals a day felt more satisfied than those who ate 5!***

In this study1

> "...researchers compared the effects of eating the same total calories divided into six meals against the effects those calories being divided into three meals....individuals who ate only three meals a day reported significantly less hunger and more satiety...the three-meals-per-day group didn't have significant drops in blood sugar, suggesting that healthy bodies, when fed right, are pretty good at self-regulation."

Similarly, we used to tell people not to miss a meal because it would slow their metabolism and they'd go into "starvation mode."

Now we know.... Lots of people are controlling their weight by practicing intermittent fasting, eating within an 8-hour window, and research indicates that going several hours without eating doesn't really affect metabolism.

Another myth that just won't go away is that people can't lose weight because "they don't eat enough." (that whole starvation thing...)

How did we ever fall for that one—have you seen a fat starving person?

With all the misinformation out there—and plenty of people willing to take your money for their advice—how do you know what to believe?

Actually, some nutrition concepts still stand the test of time:

- To lose weight, take in fewer calories than you expend.
- Eat food as unprocessed as possible.
- Build your meals around vegetables.

These 3 simple rules are the "big rocks" of a healthy diet.

PORTION PSYCHOLOGY–USE
IT TO YOUR ADVANTAGE

If you're watching your weight, manipulating your portions is a simple way to make a big difference.

It's good to know that if you serve people more food, they'll eat more.1

Scientists randomly assigned 277 people to be served a lunch with either a larger (440-calorie) or smaller (220-calorie) portion of quiche. The next day, the participants were told to serve themselves a portion from a full, family-sized quiche. (The researchers pretended that the study had some other purpose.)

People who had gotten the larger serving on day one served themselves a larger portion on day two. What's more, they also chose a larger serving when asked to identify a "normal" portion of quiche that day or a week later.

Which matters more—the size of each food item or the number of items?2

Researchers offered 186 people a plate of brownies to eat while watching a video. Each plate held 1, 2, 4, or 8 brownie squares in one of three sizes: ¼ oz., ½ oz., or 1 oz.

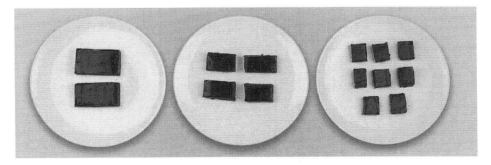

People tended to eat more when the plate held a smaller number of large brownies than when it held a larger number of small brownies.

Sixty percent of the participants ate two 1 oz. brownies, but only 40% ate four ½ oz. brownies and a mere 18% ate eight ¼ oz. brownies (even though each of the three plates held 2 oz. of brownies).

Want to eat less? Stick with smaller-size items.

3 TRICKS FOR TREATING— STRATEGIES FOR DEALING WITH HALLOWEEN CANDY

You might be surprised how often a client has told me, "I have to buy more Halloween candy. I ate most of it already." One client said she'd eaten a whole bag of Hershey's Kisses she'd bought for Halloween... at one sitting....

There are basically two kinds of people, when it comes to being around food--Abstainers and Moderators.

Moderators can decide not to eat something, or to only have one bite and have no trouble walking away.

Abstainers feel like they can't have "just one" and once they start eating something (typically that has a lot of sugar), they can't stay out of it.

If you're a Moderator, you can treat yourself to that bite-sized Snickers bar and be done.

If you're an Abstainer....

1. **Buy your least favorite candy:** Do they still make Circus Peanuts? Those things were awful! Seriously, if you're a nuts fan, buy hard candy--kids seem to like sugary candy like lollipops better anyway. If you become more discriminating, some candy won't seem good enough to be tempting. I have no trouble staying away from Hershey's chocolate, now that I've tasted the difference between "good chocolate" and "cheap chocolate."

2. **Wait until the last minute to buy candy:** Wait until Halloween day or the night before to get your treats, then store them out of sight until time for

trick-or-treaters. Keep the candy in a bowl by the door and spend the evening in another room until trick-or-treaters arrive.

3. **Get rid of it:** Donate or give away leftover candy. Keep it in the freezer, out of sight, until you dispose of it. Or if you have a lot left over, as I did last year, squirrel it out of sight in the freezer for next year.

If you still struggle with having sweets around, remember that you don't have to give out candy. There are lots of non-food options, too.

Just be sure to have your strategy in place well before October 31!

6 CHANGES I MADE TO FINALLY LOSE THOSE STUBBORN POUNDS

When you live in stretchy clothes, as I do, it's easy for weight to creep up unnoticed. Back in the spring, I had to get dressed up and struggled to get my pants to button. When I stepped on the scale, I was shocked to see I'd gained 9 pounds over my (what I considered to be) ideal weight.

I was on a mission to lose it. It had never been hard before, once I set my mind to it.

This time was different. I refused to buy into the idea that "it's harder to lose weight after a certain age." But weeks went by and that stubborn weight just wouldn't budge. I was SO frustrated.

Yesterday, I stepped on the scale and saw that I'm only 1 pound from my goal and 3 pounds from that "ideal weight." Here's what I discovered.

- **Weight loss takes more time than you might think.** I wasn't looking for a quick fix. There were days I might have bought in.... but I knew I had to change the habits that had gotten me where I was or I'd end up back where I started. Habit change doesn't yield quick weight loss. One of my mantras is "Better to do it right than do it over." Patience is lost so much faster than weight.

- **Home cooking can make a big difference.** That simply meant cooking one dish on Sundays, a casserole or soup, that I could eat the rest of the week. It's the best way to know exactly what you're eating. I still supplemented with Trader Joe's prepared salads, generally for lunch. If I did get carry-out, unless it was low calorie, I created a practice of not finishing it and putting a portion away for later.

- **Intermittent fasting is a good option for me.** Confining my eating to an 8-hour window works for me on a lot of levels--saves time in the morning, keeps my life more simple, and cuts out some calories. I eat at 11 or 12 and avoid eating past 7:30. It's not for everyone, but it works for me and has taught me....

- **It's ok to be hungry.** Most of the time it's a momentary feeling that passes, especially when I'm busy. My parents always "ate defensively" and I learned to eat because I "might get hungry." Turns out, getting hungry is ok. It's one of many things in life that can be momentarily uncomfortable toward a greater good--food tastes better when you're hungry! Lots of people have blood sugar or other issues and so I acknowledge that all situations are different.

- **The scale is simply a tool and not a judgement.** I started to weigh daily and track my weight. Weighing every day helps put that number in perspective. You can see trends within the daily fluctuations, whereas if you weigh weekly, you might measure a "low" one week and a "high" the next week. I know some people let the number dictate whether today will be a good day or a bad day. I used to be one of those people. But I learned to see the daily numbers as part of a bigger picture so each weigh-in had less power over me. If I'd been weighing every day, I never would have let myself put on those 9 pounds in the first place!

- **Light ginger beer works for me as a wine substitute.** Lots of information has been coming out about how women should have no more than 5 oz of wine per day, so I had been rethinking my wine consumption--which was always more than 5 ounces....Enter the ginger beer. One of the small bottles has 38 calories and no alcohol. I add a splash of lime sparkling water, pour it over a lot of ice and voila'! A drink I enjoy as much as the wine, that's probably saving me 300 calories. It's FeverTree Refreshingly Light Ginger Beer, in case you're interested.

You'll notice I didn't change anything about my exercise routine.

I was simply eating too many calories--easy to do when you're a small person!

THE COST OF BEING LEAN

I recently reviewed the InBody scan we had just done on a client.

This woman is strong and healthy. Her body fat percentage was 32% at her weight of 140 pounds. Losing just a little fat or adding more muscle could give her a healthier body composition.

Her reaction was, "I just wish I could get down to 115 pounds." It was time for the "How badly do you want it?" talk.

WHAT'S THE PRICE OF GETTING REALLY LEAN?1

Celebrities and social media influencers showing off their "6-pack abs" and bikini bodies create an image that their followers try to achieve-- generally to great frustration.

They don't realize that those perfect bodies don't usually stay at that level for long and they come at a price that most people aren't willing to pay.

An unhealthy body fat range is 20% and over for men and 30% and over for women. People in this category are considered "*Obese.*" Contributors to body fat in these ranges include eating processed foods, eating big portions, eating quickly, and getting no exercise.

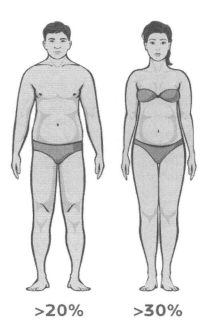

>20%   >30%

It's not too hard to move from an unhealthy range into a healthy range. Get more sleep, do some exercise, eat more unprocessed food. Essentially, it's about becoming more mindful of your habits and choosing the healthy options.

Simply making those choices results in better health, more energy, longer life expectancy, and reduced risks of metabolic syndrome. It's also possible to eliminate the need for many prescription medications.

At this level, considered "*Acceptable*," you'll look good but not super lean. Practices for staying at this level include eating slowly until satisfied at most meals, eating protein and vegetables at 1-2 meals each day, and fewer desserts and processed foods. You'll also need to sleep at least 7 hours each night and exercise 3-5 times a week at any intensity level.

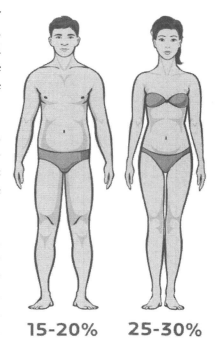

15-20%   25-30%

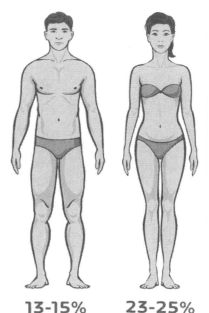

13-15%   23-25%

The trade-off is having more energy, better sleep, and finding exercise easier, and therefore more enjoyable.

This body fat level is considered "*Healthy*." Nutrition is more dialed in at this level. Practice eating slowly until satisfied at 75% of your meals. Two to three meals should have one to two servings of protein and vegetables. You'll be able to eat desserts or processed foods and drink caloric beverages 3-5 times a week.

Nutrition now requires some planning and can affect social activities.

Exercise 30-45 minutes daily with 1-2 sessions breaking a sweat and get at least 7 hours of sleep.

At this level, people reduce or eliminate many medications.

People at this level, called "*Fitness*," look very trim. To maintain it, expect to eat slowly until satisfied at 90% of your meals, all of which should include 1-2 servings of protein, vegetables, and some healthy fats.

Desserts, processed foods, and caloric beverages are limited to 1-2 times a week.

Exercise 45-60 minutes daily, with 3-4 sessions breaking a sweat, and sleep 7-8 hours a night.

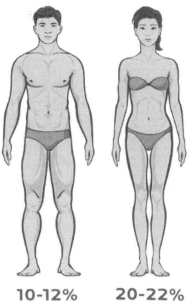

10-12%   **20-22%**

Staying at this level requires more time planning nutrition and exercising, but people often find they have fewer food cravings because of the balanced nutrition and exercise regime.

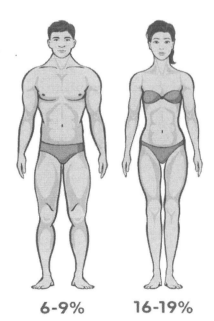

6-9%   **16-19%**

This is the "6-pack abs" level. Most Olympic athletes are in this category, called, "*Athletes*."

At this level, you would eat slowly until satisfied at 95% of your meals. Each meal would have 1-2 servings of protein, vegetables, and healthy fat. Carbs get reserved for post-workout or special training days.

Desserts, processed foods, and caloric beverages are limited to every 1-2 weeks.

Exercise 60-75 minutes daily, with 4-5 sessions breaking a sweat.

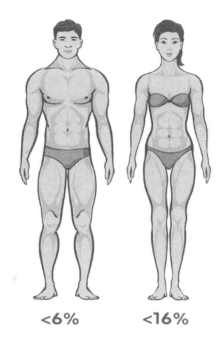

<6%   **<16%**

The *"Essential Fat"* level is considered to be unhealthy and difficult to sustain. Bodybuilders, figure competitors, and some celebrities get to this level and stay just long enough to compete or perform.

It requires eating slowly until satisfied 99% of the time, following a strict diet, sleeping 8-9 hours a night, and exercising 45-75 minutes a day, with 6-7 breaking a sweat. Desserts/processed foods are limited to once every 10-12 weeks and caloric beverages are to be avoided.

It's hard to have a social life unless you're socializing with people who share this lifestyle.

At this low body fat level, women usually stop having their period, which has significant health consequences. The focus on food and exercise can become obsessive and lead to disordered eating.

Sometimes we wistfully think about the weight we'd like to reach or return to. It's all about making choices about what we value more--our current lifestyle or the one we would need to follow to get to that goal...and stay there.

The best news is that the transition into a *healthy* range really doesn't take pain and sacrifice and the benefits of having greater mental and physical health make it worth it!

BETTER HEALTH

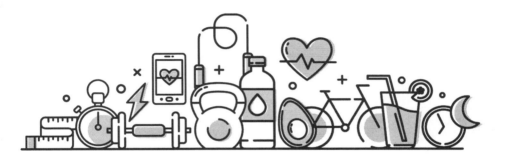

HEALTHY LIFESTYLE

THE SMARTER WAY TO WALK?
HINT...IT'S NOT HEEL/TOE

What do these things have in common?

- knee pain

- hip pain

- back pain

- bunions

- plantar fasciitis

- piriformis syndrome

- sciatica

- shoulder pain

- neck pain

- shin splints

If you guessed, "**These are all problems that can be caused by the way you walk**," you're right!

We've been told that the proper way to walk is "heel/toe" but that's a myth that probably developed when we started to wear shoes whose heels were so built up that we no longer felt them pounding the ground.

Watch people walk barefoot or notice how children walk and run and you'll see that they don't land on their heels.

Heel striking overworks the lower leg, leading to shin splints,

- hyperextends the knee joint,
- tightens the hip flexors, which pulls on the low back, drawing the "torso down" and limiting shoulder range of motion,
- causes the pelvis to rotate forward, which causes the hips to rotate inward.

This inward rotation collapses the arches, leading to bunions and potentially irritating the sciatic nerve....

There's a cascading effect throughout the body. And that's why we teach people to

- get their body straight, lifting the head and neck
- turn their feet straight ahead
- land mid-foot, center of gravity over the forward foot
- shorten their stride

Old habits can take some effort to change and re-learning how to move naturally takes a little practice.

But it can be done—I can speak from my own experience. I used to get shin splints when I walked long distances, particularly sight-seeing on vacation trips. I have never had another episode since I changed how I walk.

Once you feel the impact and pain reduction of "walking smarter," you realize that making the effort to change is worth it!

DOES SOMEONE YOU KNOW HAVE "FISH-EYE KNEES"?

Knee pain can be scary.

We hear so much about ligament and meniscus tears that when people feel knee pain they often fear the worst — surgery. The pain can be the result of a fall or other accident but more frequently it's the result of wear and tear.

Generally, when women have knee pain, it's because their hip muscles are weak, allowing the hip to collapse in, and consequently putting uneven pressure on the knee.

Men, on the other hand, often have knee pain because their knee-caps have shifted to the *outside*, called "Fish-eye Knees." In every case I've seen, these men had been athletic in their youth and it seems that muscle tightness had caused the knees to turn out.

But lately I've become aware of another factor--the way men SIT!

In every case I've seen of Fish-eye Knees, the men habitually sit with their knees apart, to the extent that many can NOT hold their knees together--no matter how hard they try.

They sit at their desk with their knees apart, drive with one knee cocked off to the side….and maybe there's a little manspreading going on there, too.

Hips and knees should line up parallel but these men **can't** stand up without splaying their knees apart!

Interestingly, when I have men with Fish-eye Knees move with their legs properly aligned, **they have no knee pain**, though some have been told they need knee replacements. In every single case, these men went to physical therapy but no one ever paid attention to how they sat or got up and down.

Here's a picture of a friend of mine that I ran across on Facebook. It perfectly illustrates the difference between men and women:

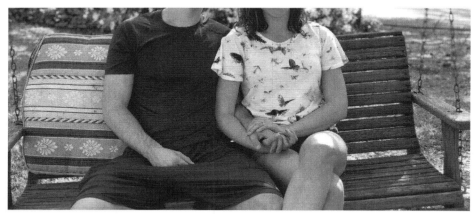

This guy is in his 20's. He's going to have some cranky knees by the time he's in his 60's.

Whether it's neck pain, shoulder pain, hip pain, back pain, knee pain, foot pain, elbow pain....there's a good chance that daily habits are contributing to the problem.

If you have something that's nagging at you, take a look at your habitual postures— it could be an issue of how you sleep, stand, walk, drive or something work related.

Changing how you move can change your life!

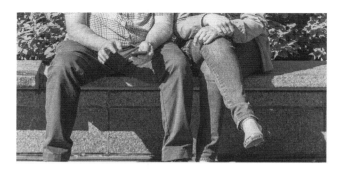

FLAT FEET? NO, YOU DON'T NEED MORE ARCH SUPPORT

Once upon a time, I was an authority on matching people with the "right" shoe for their particular needs. That was before I learned how ineffective it is to expect a shoe to do what your muscles should be doing. I had a closet full of arch supports and wore orthotics for plantar fasciitis, knee pain, iliotibial band pain, and Lord knows what all else. That was before I learned how ineffective it is to expect a shoe to do what your muscles should be doing. About 15 years ago, I got rid of them. Cold turkey.

It's exciting to see that approach becoming widely accepted. Even *Runner's World* has adopted this position.1

> "The internet and your local running store will likely urge you to buy a shoe with more arch support. Experts in the field of sports injury will instruct you to do the opposite. So who do you trust? ...the optimal shoe for you largely depends on your gait cycle, range of motion, and individual foot, among other factors."

FLAT FEET OR FALLEN ARCHES?

> "Some runners have anatomically flat feet, and other runners have what's known as 'collapsed arches,' which are flat because of a muscle weakness. Although the two types can look very similar, how you approach buying shoes for them varies widely...
>
> ...with an anatomically flat foot, arch support just sends stress up into the knee where it can lead to knee problems. That's why it's import-

ant to know what type of flat foot you have before you settle on a shoe—and take into account not just your foot but your entire body, including knees, hips, and range of motion."

We have not yet found anyone who needed arch supports because of collapsed arches. Once alignment improves and muscles get stronger, the pressure is off the arches and they come back up.

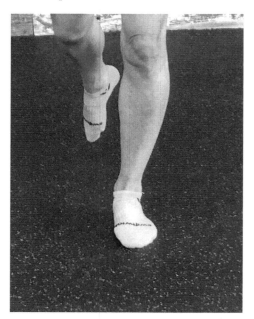

See how the arch collapses, followed by the ankle, followed by the knee?

ON OVERPRONATION AND ARCH SUPPORT

"Runners with flat feet tend to overpronate, which is when the arches of the foot roll inward after landing. (However...there are plenty of flat-footed runners who are biomechanically sound and efficient, and don't experience any overpronation.) ... Dr. Davis says people with flat feet often have really flexible feet that never get rigid for the push-off. 'The footwear industry tries to solve that by putting an arch support in there to give them an arch or create supination in the foot. **But that foot is structurally built that way, it's not something you can solve with a shoe.'**

A FULL-CONTACT MIDSOLE

"Jay Dicharry...agrees arch support can be detrimental because the arch is by nature dynamic, and having extra structure there can stop your foot from moving.

Dicharry says flat-footed runners should put more focus on seeking out a shoe with a straight 'last,' which is the mold that dictates the shape of the shoe.

A straight-lasted shoe has a wider midfoot base and less of a cut-in, a profile that has fallen by the wayside in favor of hourglass-shaped shoes... 'The problem is all these hourglass shoe shapes look nice on the wall, but when someone with a flat foot puts weight on one, part of their foot is bearing weight on the fabric upper,' he says."

When the hip muscles aren't functioning as they should, they allow the hip to internally rotate and all of your weight comes down on the arch and collapses it. That can lead to hip pain, knee pain, bunions, sciatica, plantar fasciitis, and iliotibial band syndrome—all issues I used to try to address with orthotics.

Arch supports are a Band-Aid that doesn't address the cause of fallen arches. And they don't allow for the natural "spring" of the arch.

Arch issues are best addressed by working on single leg exercises and hip strengthening, along with evaluating how you walk and run.

Once the muscles are strong, in all but the most unusual cases, you don't need that Band-Aid.

FEEL BETTER AND LOOK YOUNGER WITH THIS SIMPLE SHIFT

Neck issues can be ....well, there's a reason that we use the expression "pain in the neck" to describe something that's painful and super annoying.

Everyday habits put a ton of stress on the neck. Studies show that we shift our head closer to the screen the longer we sit in front of the computer. Most people hold their phone down and look down when texting. And I have had lots of clients who are voracious readers, tilting their head down to read, sometimes for hours on end.

Car and airplane seats are the WORST. It's nearly impossible to sit upright in them. Some occupations are harder on the neck--dentists and hair dressers are particularly vulnerable.

Then there's the psychological component--people who are depressed or don't feel well tend to hold their head down.

This "forward head" position creates neck pain because it forces little neck muscles to do the work of holding onto your head, rather than the head being balanced on your body.

It also reduces range of motion, so you can't turn your head as well--important when driving. I once had a client whose forward head position almost caused him to give up driving altogether because he couldn't look around to back up his car.

And, shoot, it just makes people look a lot older!

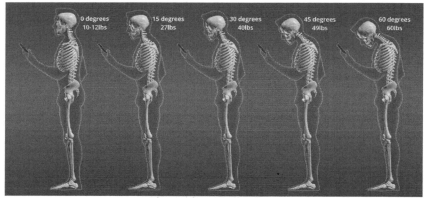

Photo credit: criticalbench.com

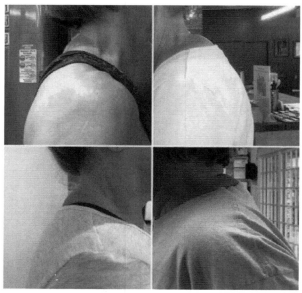

Along with this alignment comes the "hump." Most people don't even know they have it.

It's correctable if you commit to working on it.

- Shift the rearview mirror in your car up so you "lengthen" yourself when you drive.

- Use your phone and computer with your chin level.

- When traveling, use a pillow (I fold a sweater or jacket) behind your upper back to keep it from sinking into the seat.

- Use a laptop stand so you don't have to tilt your head down to use your keyboard.

- Prop pillows in your lap to hold your book up when you read.

- Raise your awareness of when you drop your head--as in situations when you feel self-conscious and want to minimize yourself. Or when you're looking over, under, or through your glasses.

- Make sure your pillows don't push your head forward at night.

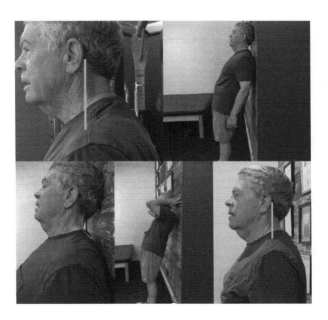

Do this exercise: https://youtu.be/rmfqPN-Cw0g

See how much difference it makes?

The sooner it's addressed, the sooner the pain can be alleviated and the greater the chance of getting rid of that hump!

THE DARK SIDE OF CORTISONE SHOTS

If you've ever had pain in your knee, hip, or even elbow, you may have had a cortisone injection in the joint. I've had them in my feet!

While cortisone can provide some relief, we're learning that the practice of injecting corticosteroids into a joint is not as safe as we thought.

Researchers at Boston University tracked 459 people and discovered an 8% complication rate with steroid injections--much higher than expected. And that number could be higher because 218 of the patients did not have follow-up imaging tests.1

Patients who received steroid shots were found to be at increased risk for:

- Accelerated OA (osteoarthritis) progression.
- Complications from death of bone in the joint, called osteonecrosis.
- Rapid joint destruction, including bone loss.
- Stress fractures that occur beneath the cartilage, known as subchondral insufficiency fracture.

Those whose X-ray findings did not show OA or only mild OA were at at higher risk for rapid worsening of their pain.

Lead research author Dr. Ali Guermazi, said his findings suggest that these injections **may do more harm than good:** steroid shots in the hips and knees may accelerate the progression of osteoarthritis and even accelerate the need for joint replacement surgeries. Evidence suggests that corticosteroid injections can be toxic to cartilage.

There are a lot of injectable options for arthritic joints, including stem cells and hyaluronic acid, but nothing has proven to provide more than short term relief.

The Arthritis Foundation recommends exercise, along with weight loss to reduce pressure on joints.

Strength training is the best preventive measure for osteoarthritis. Stronger muscles support the joints and keep them well aligned. Movement keeps joints well lubricated.

And better alignment will slow or stop the process of degeneration.

SO YOU HAD AN MRI....SLOW DOWN BEFORE YOU FREAK OUT

Eric Cressey recently shared this photo on Instagram. See how there's no space between the bones in the knee? This person *should* have knee pain.

But Cressey (a sports physical therapist) makes the point that **you can have diagnostic imaging that looks like a train wreck and have no pain.**

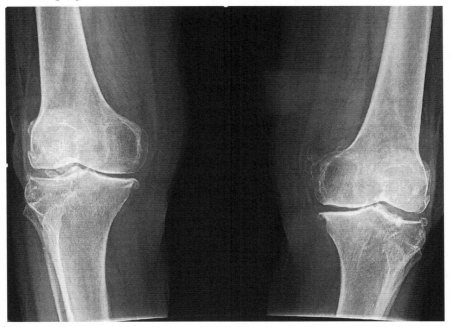

A 2010 study examined 1,862 knees and found that 36% had full-thickness cartilage tears but 14% of those had no symptoms. The researchers concluded that, "Over one-half of asymptomatic athletes have a full-thickness defect."

Another researcher looked at 268 knee tendons in basketball players. While 7% were symptomatic, 26% had degenerative changes that "should" have been painful.

Cressey says,

> "In other words, **for every one that actually presents clinically with symptoms, more than three go undiagnosed because people either haven't reached threshold, or they move well enough to keep symptoms at bay.**

> On the "move well enough" side of things...athletes with asymptomatic patellar tendinopathy actually land differently – both in terms of muscle recruitment and sequencing – than asymptomatic athletes without tendinopathy. **Fix that movement pattern and strengthen folks in the right places, and those issues never reach threshold. Leave it alone, and it's just a matter of time until they present with knee pain.**

> ....You'll see loads of chronic ACL and meniscus tears that folks never realize they have. The take-home message? Yet again, **diagnostic imaging is just one piece of the puzzle, and how you move matters just as much (if not more).**"

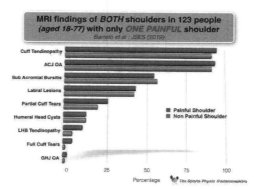

MRI says shoulders are in virtually the same condition but only 1 hurts.

Over 50% of people over 60 have rotator cuff tears, based on MRI studies.

Most of us have had a "bulging disc" and never knew it.

Dr. Jim Andrews, the renowned orthopedist and founder of Andrews Sports Medicine clinic, wrote a memorable article a few years ago, taking orthopedists to task for their reliance on imaging tests.

He referred to the unreliability of MRIs and challenged doctors to get back to looking at the patient, listening and feeling for signs and symptoms.

I've had clients who've heard some awful MRI results who've turned out to be fine---without having surgery. A lot depends on what you do with that information. MRI is just one piece of the diagnostic package.

Here's to no more test anxiety!

IS IT TIME TO PUT AWAY THE ICEPACK?

Most of us keep an icepack in the freezer, ready for bumps and bruises. On a much larger scale, cryotherapy facilities started popping up a few years ago. There, you can stand inside a tube for 2-3 minutes as your entire body gets chilled to as low as -284 degrees.

But does icing do more harm than good? This article in *Men's Health* may be bad news for the cryotherapy business.1

> "....no piece of published, peer-reviewed research has shown definitively that ice is beneficial to the healing process....recent studies have shown the opposite. Ice can delay healing, increase swelling, and possibly cause additional damage to injured tissues. That should stop you cold."

Gabe Mirkin, the doctor who created the acronym, REST--rest, ice, compression and elevation--now says, "My RICE guidelines have been used for decades, but new research shows rest and ice actually delay healing and recovery."

Ice can numb the pain.

> "But be warned: the pain will return once the tissue rewarms and the inflammatory response resumes. That's because the inflammatory response needs to happen. The three stages of healing for soft tissue injuries are... inflammation, repair and remodeling. And you can't reach the repair and remodeling phases until you've gone through Phase One."

The inflammatory response involves the production of proteins that are required for muscle healing.

> "Ice delays this process by constricting blood vessels and allowing less fluid to reach the injured area...narrowing of blood vessels caused by icing persists after cooling ends and the resulting restriction of blood flow can kill otherwise healthy tissue; that is, icing causes more damage on top of the existing injury....

> ...when ice is applied for a prolonged period, lymphatic vessels become more permeable, causing a backflow of fluid into the interstitial space. That means *local swelling...will increase*, not decrease, with the use of ice."

I used to run with people who'd finish a winter run with a plunge in the pool. They didn't know...

> "...cold water immersion after training — ice baths — substantially reduces long-term gains in muscle mass and strength by stunting the cell activity crucial for building stronger muscles. When you hit the cold tub after hard exercise, thinking you are reducing inflammation, you're actually delaying recovery."

How, then, does the body clear swelling? Muscle contraction is needed to move the fluid through the lymphatic system.

That makes me think of my numerous ankle sprains years ago. I learned that if I kept moving immediately after I twisted my ankle, it recovered faster.

> "Do you think our hunter-gatherer ancestors rolled their ankles, dug some ice out of a snowbank, sat down and stopped chasing dinner? It's more likely that they forged on, and the movement facilitated healing... a 1999 study...showed that loading damaged tissue..accelerates healing of bone and muscle tissue, while inactivity promotes aberrant tissue repair."

If an injury is too painful or fragile to move, another way to get the muscles moving is with an electric stimulation device (a.k.a. "e-stim" or TENS units. You can find them on Amazon). These low level muscle contractions help move the swelling out. Normatec boots are also effective in creating compression and systematically contracting to move swelling up from the lower extremities.

Kelly Starrett, a physical therapist who consults with TRX and Crossfit, supports ditching the ice protocol.

> "...seven years ago, he had a patient who had just had reconstructive ACL surgery. *He rehabbed the injury with no ice at all,* instead using an electrostim device. 'We had no swelling 24 hours post-surgery,' Starrett recalls. ...his patient's range of motion and quadriceps control, which often take weeks to regain after ACL reconstruction, were restored almost immediately. And because there was no swelling, there was no pain. 'We have to allow the body to excel at what it does automatically, which is heal. If you're icing, you're getting in the way, not facilitating.'"

Why do doctors and therapists still use ice?

> "Because they always have, speculates Chip Schaefer, the Chicago Bulls' director of performance health says." In the mid-90s... it was considered progressive to put ice on every player's knees after practices and games. But not anymore."

If you'd like to geek out further on the subject, check out Iced!: The Illusionary Treatment Option. available on Amazon.

And this podcast "To Ice or Not to Ice?" with Gary Reinl.

Keep moving!

BABYING YOUR BACK ACTUALLY DELAYS HEALING

The words "bulging disc" or "herniated disc" often strike terror in the hearts of back sufferers.

Those with back pain used to be advised to take to their bed. I remember my mom lying on the couch for 3 weeks after picking up two tubs of squash at the same time.

But the latest philosophy is that babying your back may delay healing.1

> "....as many as 80% of adults report at least one episode of back pain.
>
> The other 20% never experience back pain at all. But it's not because their spines are normal. Imaging tests on these pain-free folks show as much degeneration in their lower spine as everyone else has....
>
> Degeneration in your spine is a natural part of aging. 'A bulging disc, in some ways, is no different than the wrinkle next to your eye,' says Dr. Rainville.
>
> Contrary to what many people believe, only rarely does back pain strike while someone is lifting something heavy or performing an intensive activity. 'In cases of new-onset disc herniation or sciatica, only 5% of people were doing anything considered heavy physical exertion, like lifting an air conditioner,' says Dr. Rainville. Those things are rare."

It's usually something simple like brushing your teeth or more often a movement that involves bending and twisting, like making the bed, that triggers the back pain event. In gyms, it's common when someone twists to lift a weight plate from a rack.

"There is no evidence that being careful will slow the process of disc degeneration down,' says Dr. Rainville. After all, being careful won't stop any other signs of aging, such as wrinkles or gray hair....

Where back pain was once viewed a nuisance to work through, today, back pain stops many people in their tracks. 'People have gotten stuck because they've been given the advice to be careful and stop moving,' says Dr. Rainville. 'This runs counter to everything that was taught for decades to the existing.'"

So, if you're experiencing back pain caused by normal wear and tear, the message is that in most cases you don't need to stop your life and wait to heal. Move your body instead.

My coach, Todd Durkin, likes to say, "Motion is lotion."

I HURT MY BACK!
5 THINGS I LEARNED
FIRST-HAND ABOUT BACK PAIN

Recently, I hurt my back, making me part of that 80% of the population who has had back pain.

I don't even have a dramatic story to go with my injury. I simply spent 6 hours *slightly* bent over, coaching clients on my iPad. Unknowingly, I didn't practice what I preach—I **bent**, I didn't **hinge**.

It was an overuse injury--a muscle strain--just like most cases of back pain. The pain was shockingly intense. Going up and down stairs was painful in a way I never imagined. I looked like a dying bug on its back, waving my arms and legs in the air as I tried to gain momentum to roll over to get out of bed.

Back pain is the second most common reason for doctor's visits, outnumbered only by upper-respiratory infections.

Most cases of back pain are NOT caused by serious conditions, but rather poor posture and poor use of the body.

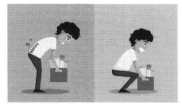

dorncompanies.com

If you haven't had back pain, there's a good chance you will. So keep this in mind:

- **Keep Moving.** Staying in the same position for a while caused the muscles to get stiff, whether I was sitting, standing, or lying down. Walking around always loosened things up and made me feel better.

- **Motrin helps and the Theragun was a God-send.** I resisted "taking something" because I thought it would only mask the pain. But in reducing the pain, it helped me move more easily, helping me move more and better. The Theragun relaxed the muscles passively and also helped keep me moving.

- **Do NOT stretch.** Muscles get strained when they're over-stretched and they get stiff because they're trying to heal. Stretching slows the whole process down and can exacerbate the injury.

- **You don't need special back exercises.** Protecting your back is about learning how to maintain good alignment, but not with a plank. You need to learn how to keep that alignment as you MOVE!

"Degenerative Disc Disease" is not a disease. It's a symptom of a spine that's taken a lot of wear and tear. You wouldn't say "Degenerative Knee Disease" would you? And if you've been told you have a "bulging disc," don't freak out. At any given time, most of us have probably had a bulging disc, and as long as it didn't press on a nerve, we wouldn't have known it. They generally resolve themselves.

Once I got past the acute couple of weeks, the pain subsided and it took a few more weeks for the stiffness to go away. I tried to be conscious of not letting my back get tucked under (losing the lumbar curve), which was how I strained it in the first place.

Interestingly, I've seen a lot of people with back pain lie on their back and draw their knees to their chest. As I can testify, that's one of the worst things you can do. Maintaining a neutral spine is the way to go.

Thanks to a very little bit of Motrin, the Theragun, and watching my alignment, I was completely back to normal in a few weeks.

Which brings me to another effective treatment….**"Tincture of Time."**

LACK OF SLEEP DRAMATICALLY RAISES YOUR RISK FOR GETTING SICK

Strep, stomach bugs, colds, flu, viruses....it's all out there and as we come together in gatherings, we're sharing a lot more than love and good will. The best ways to prevent getting sick include hand washing, not touching your face, and avoiding being around sick people. (You can forget Vitamin C and Airborne. They haven't been proven to do anything.) But there's one thing you may have missed1 "If you want to stay healthy, skip sleep at your own risk. According to the results of a new study, people who slept six hours a night or less were four times as likely to get sick after being exposed to the cold virus compared with those who got more sleep."

The researchers took 164 healthy people and monitored how much they slept. They they injected live cold viruses into their nose, quarantined them in a hotel, and waited to see who got sick.

> "How many hours a person slept, it turns out, was one of the strongest predictors of whether or not they got sick—even more than other factors like a person's age, body mass, stress levels or emotional state. People who slept six hours a night or less were four times as likely to develop a cold compared to people who slept more than seven hours a night. Those who got less than five hours of sleep a night were at 4.5 times that risk.

> When we don't sleep enough, our internal environment shifts to make us less effective at fighting off a virus... studies have shown that important immune cells are increased in the blood, meaning they're not where we really need them to be—in the immune organs like the lymph nodes—to effectively fight off viruses."

That's just one more of the many reasons we need to make getting enough sleep a priority. Try getting more sleep during the cold and flu season and see if you stay healthier.

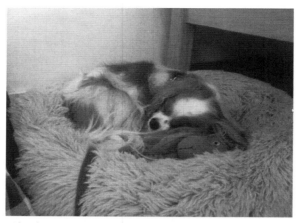

Charlie says it works for him. He's never had a cold.

THE BEST SLEEPING POSITION IS....

More and more, we're learning how important it is to sleep well. Among other things, sleep is critical to the immune system, brain function, cardiovascular health...and *lack of sleep causes you to gain weight.*

Matthew Walker says that sleep loss can even cause loneliness. "Lack of sleep induces critical changes within the brain, altering behaviour and emotions, while also disturbing essential metabolic processes and influencing the expression of immune-related genes..... people who are sleep-deprived avoid social interaction."1

THE EFFECT OF SLEEPING POSITIONS

Snoring

People snore for a lot of reasons, including allergies/nasal/sinus issues, excess weight, sleep apnea, and alcohol.

You're more likely to snore when you sleep on your back--and people who snore have worse sleep quality than those who don't.

A 1983 study consistently showed that poor sleepers sleep on their backs. In that position, as the body relaxes, the tongue can fall backward, blocking the airway and causing reduced oxygen uptake. That partially blocked airway causes the snoring sound.2

> "Recent studies have shown that in kids, snoring is always significantly associated with poor academic performance.... day time sleepiness, hyperactivity, and restless sleep were all significantly more common in snorers."

Glymphatic System Function

Researchers have only recently discovered that there is a "cleaning system" unique to the brain, called the glymphatic system. While you're sleeping, the brain is clearing itself of biological waste products--including β-amyloid plaques, the proteins that have been associated with Alzheimer's disease.

The glymphatic system works only when you're asleep.

> "As a matter of fact, it has been proven that beta amyloid accumulates during the day and can be the primary reason for many of the neurodegenerative diseases such as Alzheimer's disease and Dementia."

Studies have associated these systems with sleeping positions. Research found that people with neurodegenerative disease spend almost twice as much time on their backs while sleeping, and a more recent one in 2015 showed that the glymphatic system is most effective in the lateral position.

The ideal sleeping position is…

It would seem to be on your left side.3

> "One hypothesis holds that right-side sleeping relaxes the lower esophageal sphincter, between the stomach and the esophagus. Another holds that left-side sleeping keeps the junction between stomach and esophagus above the level of gastric acid.....scientists recruited a group of healthy subjects and fed them high-fat meals on different days to induce heartburn. Immediately after the meals, the subjects spent four hours lying on one side or the other as devices measured their esophageal acidity. Ultimately, the researchers found that "the total amount of reflux time was significantly greater" when the subjects lay on their right side."

So now, the question is "How do you maintain that position?"

We change positions an average of 35 times per night.

Sweet dreams!

3 WAYS YOU'RE AFFECTED BY SLEEP THAT YOU MIGHT NOT KNOW

Last Tuesday was a long day. I didn't sleep well the night before Katie's surgery. Honestly, I hadn't slept well for a long time, anxious about my girl. Then after the surgery, it was 1 am Wednesday before I got to bed.

Wednesday, I was a mess on 5 hours of sleep. I couldn't think straight, couldn't remember anything, and on top of that, couldn't get enough to eat.

Interestingly, *my resting heart rate was elevated, too.*

The world is full of people who function on little sleep but the evidence is clear that good quality sleep--and enough of it--is critical to good health.

YOUR BRAIN CLEANS ITSELF DURING SLEEP.

During deep sleep, your brain washes itself with cerebrospinal fluid, washing away plaques that are associated with Alzheimer's disease.

LACK OF SLEEP INCREASES HEART ATTACK RISK.1

Researchers studied 461,000 people between the ages of 40-69 who had never had a heart attack and followed them for seven years.

> "Those who slept fewer than six hours nightly were 20% more likely to have a heart attack during the study period than those who slept 7 to 8 hours a night....The risk for heart attack increased the farther people fell outside of the 6 to 9-hour optimum range. Those clocking just five hours of shuteye per night had a 52% higher risk than those

who got 7 to 8 hours a night. Long sleepers who slumbered 10 hours each night were twice as likely to have a heart attack."

Super cool news: People genetically predisposed to heart disease reduced their risk of heart attack by 18% if they slept 6-9 hours a night.

GETTING ENOUGH SLEEP HELPS WITH WEIGHT MANAGEMENT 2

- When you're sleep-deprived, you're more likely to crave junk food and your tired brain struggles with making rational choices. ..."the sleep-deprived people wanted foods that contained on average 600 calories more than what they craved when they were well rested." Just losing sleep over a few nights can cause weight gain.

- Lack of sleep affects your hormone levels--the level of ghrelin, which increases your appetite, goes up and the level of leptin, the "I've had enough" hormone, goes down.

- People who are tired from lack of sleep are less likely to exercise and be active.

- Getting enough sleep supports weight loss efforts. "A 2014 study of women ages 25 through 65 who were classified as overweight or obese and participated in a seven-month weight-loss intervention showed that women who had fragmented sleep and woke up five or more times a night lost less weight than the women who had higher-quality sleep."

We know that it's better to set a routine in which you go to bed and get up at the same times each day--even on weekends.

Make sure the room is dark and not too warm. Avoid anything stimulating before bed, whether it's caffeine or a suspenseful movie.

And be sure you've moved enough during the day to be tired at night.

VISCERAL FAT—THE #1 PREDICTOR OF DISEASE
Here's A Quick Way To Measure Yours

All fat is not the same. There's essential, subcutaneous, and visceral fat.

Essential is what you might expect--fat that is necessary for good health. Subcutaneous fat is below the skin--the "pinch an inch" fat. When you think of Santa Claus's belly "that shook like a bowl full of jelly"--that's subcutaneous fat.

Then, there's visceral fat, found inside the abdominal cavity, around your organs. Visceral fat is under the muscle. People with a lot of visceral fat have a firm belly, regardless of its diameter. It's possible to have visceral fat AND subcutaneous abdominal fat.

Endocrinologist Robert Lustig says in his book, Fat Chance,1

"Visceral fat is the fulcrum on which your health teeters.

When it comes right down to it, it's all about your middle. This whole obesity/health/longevity question centers on your abdominal, visceral, or 'big belly' fat .....In a nutshell, your body fat is your biggest long-term risk for infirmity. Nothing correlates with diabetes, heart disease, and cancer better than your fat."

Is your visceral fat level too high?

A simple way to measure is your waist-to-height ratio. The optimal ratio is <.5. A waist measurement of more than 40 inches for men and 35 inches for women is a likely indicator of visceral fat.

Visceral fat deposits are hormonally driven. That's why men usually carry their fat in the abdomen and women's fat deposits shift from the extremities to the abdomen in the wake of the loss of estrogen post-menopause.

That's when heart disease risks for women rise.

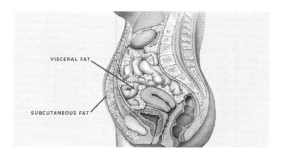

The simplest and cheapest way to determine your health status is your waist circumference, which correlates with morbidity and risk for death better than any other health parameter. This is arguably the most important piece of information in your entire health profile because it tells you about your visceral fat. A high waist circumference translates into the "apple shape" that tips physicians off to risk for diabetes, heart disease, stroke, and cancer.

My dad was 5'8" and his waist size ranged from 42 to 44 inches. His ratio would be .67. He died of cancer at the young age of 72. Granted, his waist measurement reflects lifestyle habits of poor food choices and inactivity.

If you're looking for a quick assessment of whether you need to lose some weight, this one's easy to calculate.

It's not just about appearance.

It's about securing your long term good health.

KEEPING YOUR MUSCLES FIT IS TIED TO BETTER HEART HEALTH

You know how critical it is to stay strong and maintain your muscle mass.

Skeletal muscle is important for staying strong and self-sufficient, but also for preventing injury, maintaining metabolic rate, and maintaining blood sugar levels, among many other things.

Low muscle mass has been correlated with cardiovascular disease--but does low muscle mass lead to heart disease or does heart disease cause disability that leads to low muscle mass?

Researchers in Greece studied more than 1000 people (who had no evidence of heart disease at the beginning of the study) over 10 years and discovered that between the beginning and end of that decade, 27% of the participants had developed heart disease. The incidence was 6 times higher in men.1

> "...people's muscle mass at the study's start was linked to their chances of heart disease now. **Those people with the most muscle then were the least likely to have heart disease now.** That association remained significant when the scientists controlled for people's diet, education and physical activity, but not when they looked at gender. Women's muscle mass was not associated with later risks for heart disease, in large part because so few of the women had developed heart disease. In general, women tend to get heart disease about 10 years later than men. But for men, **having relatively large amounts of muscle early in middle age dropped the risk of heart disease later by 81 percent...**"

People who have relatively more muscle are likely to be more active, so that could explain part of the decreased heart disease risk. BUT the researchers speculate that the contributions muscle makes to blood sugar control and decreasing inflammation are major factors.

Keep in mind, we can only speculate the effect on women, because they generally get heart disease later in life. Given their hormonal shifts post-menopause, it's reasonable to expect the same effect, just a little later.

Protect that ticker by staying fit and active. It's never too early or too late to start to see improvements in your health and quality of life.

WHEN IT COMES TO DEPRESSION, EXERCISE CAN TRUMP GENETICS

People frequently refer to a wide array of issues that "run in my family." *We're learning that genes are not necessarily our destiny and lifestyle habits can often mitigate genetics.*

Case in point: A new study found that "almost any type of physical activity, whether strenuous or light, helped to offset people's genetic propensity for depression, though the benefits were greater when people exercised more often." [1]

Depression is considered to have a genetic component but exercise has been linked to shortening bouts of depression and higher aerobic fitness is associated with lower risk.

In the new study, which was published in *Depression* and *Anxiety*, researchers asked almost 8,000 people about their exercise habits and noted their medical records and genetic risks for depression.

People who were genetically predisposed to depression were more likely to develop it, but [2]

> "... physically active people had less risk than people who rarely moved, and the type of exercise barely mattered. If someone spent at least three hours a week participating in any activity, whether it was vigorous, such as running, or gentler, like yoga or walking, he or she was less likely to become depressed than sedentary volunteers, and the risk fell another 17 percent with each additional 30 minutes or so of daily activity."

The risk of subsequent bouts of depression dropped for those who started exercising. And *people with a genetic risk for depression were no more likely to develop depression than inactive people with little genetic risk.*

"In effect, physical activity neutralized much of the added risk for people born with a propensity for depression, says Karmel Choi, a clinical and research fellow at Massachusetts General Hospital and Harvard's T.H. Chan School of Public Health...

The findings also underscore that genes are not destiny, Dr. Choi says. If depression runs in your family, she says, you might help to manage any heightened risk by moving more."

We learn more all the time about how intricately the mind and body are intertwined.

"THE KEY TO A LONG LIFE HAS LITTLE TO DO WITH 'GOOD GENES'"

My friend Phil and I go round and round on this subject. He thinks that longevity comes down to genetics, while having observed my family's history and habits, I just don't buy it.

Turns out, *longevity has a familial association not related to genetics.*

A group of researchers sifted through over 400 million people in Ancestry.com's archives and concluded that1

> "...**although longevity tends to run in families, your DNA has far less influence on how long you live than previously thought**....' The true heritability of human longevity for that cohort is **likely no more than seven percent**,' says Ruby. Previous estimates for how much genes explain variations in lifespan have ranged from around 15 to 30 percent."

Here's where it really gets interesting.

> "...through every generation, people are much more likely to select mates with similar lifespans than random chance would predict.... you might choose a partner who also has curly hair, and if the curly-haired trait winds up being somehow associated with long lifespans, this would inflate estimates of lifespan heritability passed on to your kids. Same thing for non-genetic traits like wealth, education, and access to good health care....

> The first hint that something other than genetics or a shared family environment might be at work came when Ruby tried looking at in-

law relatives. ...They investigated parent-child pairs, sibling pairs, various cousins, and so on. Nothing much surprising popped out there.

But when Ruby looked at in-laws, things started to get weird. Logic suggests you shouldn't share significant chunks of DNA with your siblings' spouse—say your brother's wife or your sister's husband.

But in Ruby's analysis, **people connected through a close relative's marriage were almost as likely to have similar lifespans as people connected through blood.** '...it aligns well with how we know human societies are structured.'

For now, the big takeaway seems to be that **humans have more control over how long they live than their genes do. It's all the other things that families share—homes and neighborhoods, culture and cuisine, access to education and health care—that make a much bigger difference in the set of numbers that might one day grace your tombstone.**

Maybe that's why Ancestry's chief scientific officer Catherine Ball says the company has no plans to offer a longevity score in any of its DNA testing products any time soon. '**Right now a healthy lifespan looks to be more of a function of the choices that we make,**' she says.

She points to places in the data where lifespans took big hits—for males during World War I, and then in two waves in the latter half of the 20th century as men and then women took up a cigarette habit.

'**Don't smoke, and don't go to war. Those are my two pieces of advice,**' she says."

If your family doesn't have a history of longevity, you can change your odds of greater longevity by making especially good choices. And if your family members tend to live a long time, don't waste that genetic fortune by making unhealthy choices.

Either way, you have more power than you might think!

SET UP YOUR COMPUTER WORKSPACE FOR LESS PAIN, MORE GAIN

Working at the computer has been linked to:

- Carpal Tunnel Syndrome

- Rotator Cuff Syndrome

- De Quervain's tendinitis

- Trigger finger

- Eyestrain

- Back Pain

Researchers have identified sitting positions that put extra stress on your back and neck:

- Sitting with the back at a 90 degree angle to the legs

- Sitting with the upper body bent forward at the waist

- Sitting with the head tilted upward (for example, to view a monitor above eye level)

- Sitting while looking down or to the side (for instance, viewing a document on the desk)

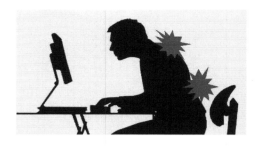

People who sit for long periods of time run a high risk of low back injury, second only to those who lift heavy weights.

Let's take a look at the optimal work station.

1. **Head** - Should be level, not tilted or twisted. The monitor should be set so that the top of the screen is at eye height--you shouldn't have to look up to see your monitor. To prevent eye strain, position the monitor as far away as possible while still being able to read it clearly. Place your reference materials and monitor at the same height, as close as possible to the same distance from your eyes, to minimize refocusing your eyes as you look back and forth between them. Your monitor should be placed at a right angle from any windows. Facing a window with your monitor in front of you creates a backlit monitor and can cause additional eyestrain.

2. **Shoulders** - Relaxed, elbows close to side, chest lifted.

3. **Back rest** - Tilted back 10 to 20 degrees, supporting the lower back with the curve of chair.

4. **Armrests** - Supporting forearms equally, keeping your arms next to your body. The height of the arms should keep wrists straight forward when working.

5. **Wrists** - Straight, in line with forearms. Be sure to keep your wrist straight when operating the mouse. If you find yourself resting the heel of your hand on the front of the keyboard or desk, your keyboard is too high.

6. **Hips** - Should fit comfortably into chair, leaving a small gap between knees and the front of the seat. Your weight should be on your "sitting bones." Be sure your "tail" isn't tucked under.

7. **Knees** - Slightly lower than hips, known as the "astronaut position." This reduces the amount of body weight your spine has to support, as the chair's backrest takes some of the load.

8. **Feet** - Flat on floor or supported by a footrest. You can get special "under the desk footrests." I use a yoga block or Charlie's bed.

LAPTOPS

It's tempting to use your laptop at a table, lying down, or propped in your lap. This convenience is why we love laptops but for using it any length of time, I swear by my laptop stand--it's better for you AND your computer--it keeps it cooler.

STANDING DESKS

I don't love standing desks because the issue is not so much standing vs sitting as an issue of movement.

Use a standing desk in blocks of 1-2 hours to avoid locking out the knees as the quads fatigue, leading to back strain and collapsed arches. Obviously, if you're going to use a standing desk, *don't wear heels*!

Follow the "Rule of 20": For every 20 minutes of computer time, take at least 20 seconds to focus on an object 20 feet away.

TAKE BREAKS

Your eyes need time to focus on far-away objects and your body needs a break to move and stretch.

Flex your arms and legs, stand up and stretch, and rotate your ankles and feet. Take these "micro-breaks" in addition to 15-minute breaks every 2 hours.

While seated at your workstation:

- Squeeze your shoulder blades together with your elbows lifted away from your body.

- Rotate your shoulders backwards with your arms relaxed at your sides. Repeat three times.

- Raise your arms above your shoulders, reaching upward.

- Clench your fists, release them, and spread your fingers wide. Hold each position for a count of three.

"FIX YOUR FEET"– BY CHANGING WHAT YOU WEAR ON THEM

The subject of choosing shoes and how to walk and run comes up all the time. After watching an evolution of "motion control" shoes, orthotics, cushioning, and "support," I now have no doubt that less is more when it comes to shoes and all the correction we were expecting to get from our shoes needs to be done from higher up in the body--most notably at the hips and pelvis.

As Brian Johnson says on his website, Optimize1…

> "We evolved for millions of years without shoes and our feet took care of business....everyone went from being barefoot or wearing moccasins or sandals to wearing big ol' overprotecting shoes.
>
> Why should we care? Because a bunch of **our biomechanical issues—from sore knees and hips and lower backs—can be traced back to sub-optimal feet.** Enter: 'Fix Your Feet' by Phil Maffetone.
>
> Maffetone tells us that **all the artificial support in sports shoes actually weakens the very feet we're trying to help out.** … Injuries that are pretty much totally preventable. And, **when we have artificial cushioning, we mess with our gait. Specifically, we tend to overstride which tends to make us have an abnormal heel strike. Which tends to lead to all the injuries we don't want."**

Quoting Maffetone:

> "A number of factors can disrupt a person's normal gait. … The most common factor that changes a normal gait to an abnormal one is wear-

ing shoes. **Most shoes, including the sports type such as the popular running shoes, change the gait by causing the stride length to be abnormally longer. This results in an abnormal heel strike—hitting the ground further back on the heel.** This is especially a problem when jogging or running because it places more shock through the foot and into the knee and occurs despite the shoe cushioning or other shoe designs.

Barefoot movement of any type does not cause the same stress. ... our feet were made for walking, running, hopping, jumping, and all other natural movements....Apart from sandals and moccasins, humans evolved barefoot—for millions of years our feet were free. Suddenly, in only the past few hundred years, shoes of many types have restricted our feet, disturbed our gait, and caused untold problems to our feet, triggering other problems throughout the body they support."

Plantar fasciitis, bunions, and a host of foot issues are relatively unknown in cultures that go barefoot.

Maffetone continues:

"....when we throw shoes on our feet that do anything more than protect the bottoms from rocks and scrapes (like those simple sandals and moccasins), we're messing around with perfection.....With the advent of today's modern shoes came a whole array of foot problems complete with companies that made therapeutic devices and professionals to treat such conditions. Many companies and individuals have benefited, as **the shoe industry and these products and services connected with the epidemic of foot problems are big business.**

Without the restriction of shoes, your foot muscles can ultimately return to their natural state of optimal function. In some people, this could take time... **if you're used to wearing high-heeled shoes or thick-soled sports shoes most of the time, being barefoot will be a big transition.** But once you experience the freedom of being bare, you'll wonder how you got by without it."

Here's where people made a big mistake. They jumped into "barefoot shoes" straight out of super cushioned or overly stabilized shoes and their body didn't have a chance to make the transition. Then **we had a rash of injuries that people**

blamed on the shoes, when they needed to change their gait mechanics and allow their body to adjust.

Johnson elaborates,

> "All that unnecessary protection...messes with our gait while weakening all the muscles that *should* be working like they've been designed to work for millions of years. Plus, shoes distribute our weight in a weird way—which leads to even more issues. The most extreme example? High-heeled shoes. ...we have a culture that puts wearing a "costume" ahead of function....."

Yep. Studies show that people burn more calories on "Casual Fridays" because their attire makes it easier for them to move--walk more steps and take the stairs. ***During Birmingham's "Snowmageddon" lots of women were trapped at work because they couldn't walk home in their high heels.***

> "In... the British Journal of Sports Medicine, researchers Robbins and Waked state, **'Expensive athletic shoes are deceptively advertised to safeguard well through 'cushioning impact' yet account for 123% greater injury frequency than the cheapest ones.'"** ~ Phil Maffetone

I've actually known people who have run in these "platform shoes" and others who "love the cushioning."

But the foot is designed to be flexible and most shoes encase that natural flexibility in an inflexible box.....or on top of a mattress...

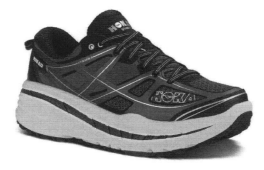

WHAT YOU DON'T KNOW
ABOUT SHOES

Shoes can be fun accessories but they can also wreck knees, hips, and the back.

Dr. William Rossi--a podiatrist--wrote "Why Shoes Make "Normal" Gait Impossible" for the journal *Podiatry Management.*1

> "Each year, consumers spend hundreds of millions of dollars for "walking shoes" promising to help the wearer walk "right" or more comfortably. Each year, additional hundreds of millions of dollars are spent for orthotics designed to "normalize" foot balance, stability, and gait. Podiatrists and other medical practitioners are constantly applying therapies and ancillary products to correct gait faults and re-establish "normal" gait. ...**natural gait is biomechanically impossible for any shoe-wearing person....in shoe-wearing societies many people have what appears to be "normal" gait, while in shoeless societies they have "natural" gait. And there are pronounced differences between the two both in form and function.**"

*People often say, "I don't wear high heels--no more than 2 inches." **Take a look at the effect of a 2" heel.***

"Does the wearing of low, one inch "sensible" heels prevent these problems of postural adaptation? No. All the low heel does is lessen the intensity of the negative postural effects. Hence, **the wearing of heels of any height automatically alters the natural erect state of the body column....**"

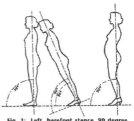

Fig. 1: Left, barefoot stance, 90 degree angle with perpendicular; center, if body column were rigid, on medium 2-inch heel angle is reduced to 70 degrees; right, to regain 90 degree angle on 2-inch heel, body column must make adjustments.

Did you know that people generally no longer use their toes when they walk?

"If you rest a shoe, new or old, on a table and view it in profile from the side, it reveals an up-tilt of the toe tip varying from five-eighths to one inch or more. More on worn shoes. This is known as "toe spring" and is built into the last. On the bare, natural foot the digits rest flat, their tips grasping the ground as an assist in step propulsion. Inside the shoe, the digits are lifted slantwise off the ground, unable to fulfill their…ground grasping function.

So why is toe spring built into the last and shoe? **To compensate for lack or absence of shoe flexibility at the ball. The toe spring creates a rocker effect on the shoe sole so that the shoe, instead of full flexing as it should, forces the foot to "roll" forward like the curved bottom of a rocking chair.** The thicker the sole, such as on sneakers or work boots, or the stiffer the sole, the greater the toe spring needed because of lack of shoe flexibility.

With toe spring, the toes of the foot are constantly angled upward five to twenty degrees, depending upon the amount of shoe toe spring... **they are 'forced out of business,'** denied much or all of their natural ground-grasping action and exercise so essential to exercising of the whole foot because 18 of the foot's 19 tendons are attached to the toes.

Why are lasts made with a concavity under the ball? Tradition. About 80 years ago, **a shoe manufacturer discovered that the foot could be made to look smaller and trimmer by allowing it to "sink" into a cavity under the ball of the foot** that no one would see—thus reducing the amount of foot volume visible above. It was so successful in its **mission of smaller-looking feet** that it was quickly adopted by other manufacturers. It has long since become a standard part of last design….a sinkhole into which the three middle metatarsal heads fall as the first and fifth heads rise on the rim.

We thus have the classic "fallen" metatarsal arch. The application of a metatarsal pad... provides relief—not because it "raises" the arch but simply by filling in the cavity and returning the heads to their natural level plane.

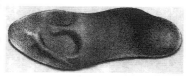

... all shoes flex 30 to 80 percent less than normal at the ball.... The foot must now work harder to take each of its approximately eight thousand daily steps. The required extra energy imposes undue strain and fatigue on the foot. Why are most shoes inflexible? First, **the average shoe bottom consists of several layers of materials or components: outsole, midsole, insole, sock liner, filler materials, cushioning. This multiple-layered sandwich poses a formidable challenge to bending or flexing.** Second, many types of footwear—athletic, sneakers, work and outdoor boots, walking, casual, etc.—have thick soles which add further to inflexibility. Many elderly people whose feet have lost elasticity and flexibility over the many years of shoe wearing have difficulty climbing or descending stairs......"

Most shoes weigh too much. The average pair of dress shoes weighs about 34 ounces... some work and outdoor boots up to 60 ounces or more. Women's dress and casual shoes average 16-24 ounces a pair; women's boots about 32 ounces. A lightweight pair of 16-ounce shoes amounts to a cumulative four tons of foot-lift load daily (16 ounces times 6,000 foot-lift steps). **If the shoes weigh 32 ounces, daily footlift load is eight tons.....**

Every added four ounces of shoe weight adds another one ton to foot-lift load. These **foot lift loads impose an energy drain not only on the foot but the whole body.....No footwear, with certain exceptions, should weigh more than 12 ounces a pair for women, 16-18 ounces for men.....**"

Your feet need to feel contact with the ground.

"The soles and tips of the toes contain over 200,000 nerve endings, perhaps the densest concentration to be found anywhere of comparable size on the body. Our nerve-dense soles are our only tactile contact with the physical world around us. Without them we would lose equilibrium and become disoriented... there is a sensory foot/body, foot/brain connection vital to body stability, equilibrium, and gait. Yet, much of it is denied us because of our thick-layered, inflexible shoes....

It took four million years to develop our unique human foot and our consequent distinctive form of gait, a remarkable feat of bioengineering. Yet, in only a few thousand years, and with one carelessly designed instrument, our shoes, we have warped the pure anatomical form of human gait, obstructing its engineering efficiency, afflicting it with strains and stresses and denying it its natural grace of form and ease of movement head to foot.

We have converted a beautiful thoroughbred into a plodding plowhorse."

What about orthotics? Podiatrists & orthopedists are still recommending them. I am one of many who used to own a closet full of various supports and haven't worn any in years--and my feet are fine.

"A secure, stable superstructure cannot be erected on a design-defective base or foundation (the Tower of Pisa is a classic example). **In regard to "restoring" natural gait, shoe and orthotic are biomechanically incompatible.**"

There is one issue that I don't see addressed--**feet were likely not designed to tolerate *standing for long periods.*** I swear by minimal soled, flexible shoes, but when I've been on my feet for 12 hours, getting home to my flexible-with-anatomical-footbed Chacos feels like heaven!

MINDSET

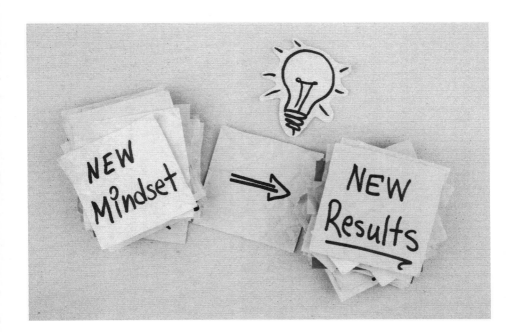

"DON'T GET AHEAD OF YOUR HEADLIGHTS..."

This morning I worked with a client who came to me 3 months ago, having been told that he needed surgery on his right shoulder by 3 orthopedists. One even went so far as to say, "There's *so much* work to be done in there, I'm not even sure the surgery can be done arthroscopically."

Fast forward to today--he did a chest press with a 20# dumbbell on that right side (and a 35# dumbbell on the left!). He said that 75% of the time he has no pain at all and feels like it gets better every week. This 76 year old man may be the strongest he's ever been.

He's not just stronger, his posture is so much straighter that I find myself thinking he looks younger. His joints move better and we're correcting issues with his left knee and gait mechanics.

He came to me because he wanted to avoid surgery and all of its implications.

Shoulder surgery is a big deal--it's the most likely surgery to lead to pain medication addiction.

He'd gotten a disturbing diagnosis, was living with pain, and fearful of what the future might hold. Now, not only is the shoulder functional, he's better in so many ways.

One of my very favorite people reminds me regularly, "**Don't get ahead of your headlights.**"

All we know is what we know NOW and speculating about tomorrow can take the joy from today. When this client was told his shoulder was in bad shape and needed surgery, he couldn't have known that diagnosis would lead him to being stronger, straighter, more fit, and actually *happier*--pain is depressing!

That scary diagnosis had a terrific outcome.

Have you ever had an injury and thought, "I'll never be able to _____ again."?

Or looked in the mirror and thought, "I'm never going to get this weight off."?

Or quit an exercise program...again...and thought, "I keep saying I'm going to get in shape but it's never going to happen!" ?

It's time to ditch that dusty crystal ball!

The key is to focus on what have control over ***today***.

I have one client who has torn the meniscus and ACL in each knee in skiing accidents, yet has come back both times to ski again. We have clients who've lost a lot of weight, after struggling with their weight for most of their lives.

Tonight I heard from a client, an avid tennis player, who tore his meniscus a year ago. At the time, it was tempting to speculate that he might never play again. But we kept doing what we knew to do and.... today he played his first time back on the court since his injury--and won!

I'm preaching to myself here, too. I freak out at IRS notices in the mail or when we lose a client. With a lot of practice, I'm getting better at not getting ahead of my headlights, as I discover how much it reduces my stress levels.

Stress management is as important to good health as eating well and getting enough sleep. Let's make a pact to leave fortune telling to the experts and live in the light of those beams.

THE BIGGEST OBSTACLE IS MINDSET ACHIEVE YOUR GOALS WITH THIS APPROACH

The world is so small these days. I was contacted recently by someone in Philadelphia who'd been referred to me--on Twitter-- by someone in Wales.....

The woman in Philly, "Desiree," was asking about her back pain but our email conversation quickly turned to her desire to lose weight--she used to weigh 130 pounds and now weighs 200 pounds.

Desiree mentioned that she was "waiting for the refrigerator to arrive" and doesn't like vegetables. I could only speculate about what she's been eating.

She asked about fasting and whether it's ok to eat non-GMO foods.

I suggested she start with *easy* changes, like ways she can increase her activity level and simple dietary swaps.

HAVE YOU HEARD OF ZENO'S PARADOX?

It's the idea that if you cover half the distance between where you are and where you want to be, you'll never get there.

Elizabeth Langer, who wrote one of my favorite books, Counterclockwise, suggests applying the opposite of Zeno's Paradox--that **we can always take tiny steps in the direction of our goals.**

Want to lose weight? Desiree wants to lose 70 pounds. That might seem overwhelming but 70 ounces is still moving in the right direction.

And steady, gradual progress is often more likely to lead to lasting change.

> As long as you keep moving in the direction of your goals, you're better off than you were before.

If you're frustrated with reaching goals you've set, set smaller goals that will move you towards your larger goal.

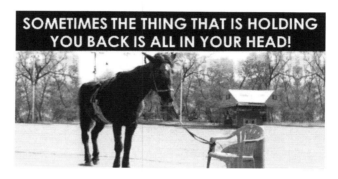

SOMETIMES THE THING THAT IS HOLDING YOU BACK IS ALL IN YOUR HEAD!

Desiree set a goal of giving up her soda habit...for a week.

What *small* changes can you make to make your life better?

I WAS ROBBED...
MAKING A MINDSET SHIFT FROM SETBACK TO COMEBACK

In July of 2019, I learned that the owner of the payroll company we used had wired money out of the company, long story short, committing wire fraud.

Three weeks later, I discovered that money from our account had not been used to pay our taxes, it was part of that stolen $122 million. (Yes, you read that right.)

The new payroll company estimated that our tax liability--what now remained to be paid--AGAIN--could amount to over $14,000.

I was heartsick. Lower than low. Some days felt like nothing was going right.

Over the course of a few days, I pulled myself out of my funk, as I thought of people who'd happily trade my problems for theirs. The situation was a nightmare, but not devastating.

I started to work on my mindset.

Jack Canfield, author of Chicken Soup For The Soul, writes:

> **"It's important to remember that you have the power to change your experience at any moment. And that's because it's your thoughts that create your own reality."**

My great lesson from reading E-Squared was that we will find in the world what we are looking for.

The things you choose to focus on determine how you perceive the world— AND the experiences you have as a result.

I remind myself, "Energy flows where your attention goes."

Here's my mindset strategy, courtesy of Jack Canfield:

1. Be Aware of Your Thoughts

Start paying attention to the things you tell yourself – and remember that you have the power to change them. Take a moment to reflect on the thoughts you were thinking. Were they positive or negative? Were they fear-based or optimistic?

2. Reframe Negative Thoughts

Whenever you find yourself thinking something like, "You can't trust other people." or "I'm never going to get good at this." or "There's no point in trying because I'll probably fail." – take the time to transform that thought into a positive one. Tell yourself: "I have such great people in my life." or "I know I'll get this if I just work at it." or "Let's give it a try. It's the only way I'll ever succeed — and even if I fail, at least I will have learned something, and I can try again."

3. Visualize Positive Outcomes

Imagine what that positive outcome will look and feel like. The more clearly you can see it in your mind, the more easily you'll make that vision a reality.

4. Develop a Daily Gratitude Practice

Spend time every day thinking about what's good in your life. The friends and family you have in your life. Your home, your job, your pet, clean water, electricity, the beauty of the natural world around you. The fact that you have clothes to wear and good food to eat. You will realize that your life is FULL of wonderful things to be thankful for. A daily gratitude practice—either writing in a journal or just speaking it out loud—makes it even easier to maintain a positive mindset.

I'm determined not to think about "the worst" because I know if that's what I'm focusing on, it's what I'll find. That won't come easy for me--I didn't grow up with positive thinkers. But I'm blessed with good health, wonderful people in my life, a strong work ethic.... and just a bit of a Pollyanna streak.

3 STRATEGIES FOR LIVING LONGER BY BECOMING AN OPTIMIST

What if you could significantly reduce your risk of cardiovascular disease—and extend your lifespan—simply by changing your outlook on life?

That's exactly what a meta-analysis of 15 studies including 229, 391 individuals suggests.1

The researchers found that those with a positive outlook enjoyed a 35% reduction in cardiovascular events and an 18% reduction in early death, compared to those with a pessimistic outlook.

These effects surpass—*significantly*—the effects that you could expect from taking statin drugs.

The researchers speculated that people who were more optimistic were more likely to engage in health-promoting behaviors, like eating well and exercising.

But there's another explanation for these benefits: neuroplasticity. Research in neuroscience over the last 30 years has conclusively shown that:

1. The brain is the control center for health.
2. Our thoughts, emotions, behaviors, and experiences change the structure and functioning of our brain.

What we think, how we feel, and how we respond to life has a direct and measurable impact on our physiology—and thus on our health and our lifespan.

We're not talking about "New Age" philosophy here.

This is based on peer-reviewed, scientific studies that have been published in some of the most reputable journals in the fields of neuroscience and neuropsychology.

Some people are pessimistic by nature or grew up in a pessimistic environment, so becoming more optimistic will take some practice.

Here are some ways to get you started...

- Jocko Willink has his "**Good**" response to EVERYTHING that ever happens to him. https://youtu.be/IdTMDpizis8. Watching this video got me through some tough times.

- Brian Johnson wrote in his Optimize blog about a way to create a mindset shift, taken from a book called *Golden Rules for Everyday Life*. 2

    "For thousands of years the pearl oyster has been there, as a lesson to human beings, but they have never understood it. And what does it teach us? Simply that, if we wrap our difficulties and all the things that annoy us in a soft, luminous, opalescent matter, we will be very rich indeed....

    *.....instead of complaining and doing nothing to stop yourself from getting worn down by your difficulties, set to work to secrete this special matter and wrap them up in it. **Every time you have to put up with a painful situation or somebody you really can't bear, be glad, and say, 'Lord God, what luck: another grain of sand, and a potential new pearl.'** If you really understand the example of the pearl oyster, you will have enough work to keep you busy for the rest of your life."*

- Oprah Winfrey has a line that I come back to again and again, "**Man's rejection is God's protection.**"

- Replacing the thought, "Why is this happening **TO** me?" with "Why is this happening **FOR** me?" has helped me so much to keep a positive outlook.

By being optimistic, we can bring more light into this world and have more years to do it!

CELEBRATE!
IT'LL MAKE YOU HAPPIER!

Celebrating something makes people happier than those who celebrate nothing.

Dan Buettner, who wrote The Blue Zones, in which he described the characteristics of the 5 areas where people live the longest, also wrote The Blue Zones Of Happiness.1

> "People from the happiest places in the world find ways to actively express their gratitude and celebrate life. In Mexico, Dan Buettner met famously happy columnist and humorist Armando Fuentes Aguirre (known as El Catón by his friends) who believes his country's high happiness scores may be connected to their culture of celebration. 'We celebrate everything. Mother's Day. Father's Day. Godfather's Day… Something every week. We invent reasons together,' Fuentes said….
>
> We know from the longest-lived people in the world that those who put family first and socialize with their friends tend to live longer, happier lives.
>
> Matthew Killingsworth… has collected data from over 20,000 people who report how happy they feel at randomly selected moments during daily life…the data reveals people are actually happier than usual on holidays.
>
> Spending time with our friends and family turns out to be a robustly positive predictor of our happiness."

That reminded me of my coping mechanism when I moved from Chapel Hill to D.C. I was so sad and lonely and missed Chapel Hill terribly. So I found everything I could to celebrate--I even had a Valentine's Day wreath. I made an extra big deal about birthdays. Christmas became an extravaganza. I celebrated everything I could--and it lifted my spirits!

Just Your WORDS Can Make You Happier!

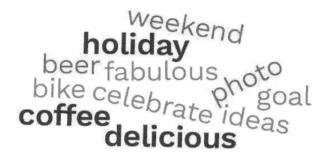

"Recent research published in PLOS ONE analyzed language patterns of volunteers on social media and found people who use words such as "weekend," "coffee," "holiday," and "delicious," score high for positive emotions." 2

Those folks who put Christmas decorations up at Halloween may be on to something.

> "We know that savoring the little things and having gratitude can lead to greater overall well-being. **Celebrating for longer may extend those positive feelings.** A study from the Journal of Environmental Psychology suggests that holiday decorations tell neighbors you're accessible and friendly, open to socializing and making new friends."3

You don't need a holiday to find something to celebrate. Just celebrating life's pleasures and blessings is enough.

"Drink without getting drunk
Love without suffering jealousy
Eat without overindulging
Never argue

And once in a while, with great discretion, misbehave."
—Armando Fuentes Aguirre, El Catón

STRESS REALLY CAN
GIVE YOU GRAY HAIR

One more reason to reduce stress? It actually does give you gray hair!

As we get older, the stem cells that produce pigment in our hair follicles gradually disappear, causing hair to lose pigment....and our hair grays.

Harvard researchers discovered that the norepinephrine produced by the nervous system when we're under stress gets into hair follicles and causes the stem cells to ultimately move out of the hair follicles. This results in new hair growing in white or gray.

They also found that stress leads to the loss of these pigment-producing stem cells in mice.

"When we started to study this, I expected that stress was bad for the body—but the detrimental impact of stress that we discovered was beyond what I imagined," says Dr. Ya-Chieh Hsu of Harvard University, who led the study. "After just a few days, all of the melanocyte stem cells were lost. Once they're gone, you can't regenerate pigments anymore. The damage is permanent."1

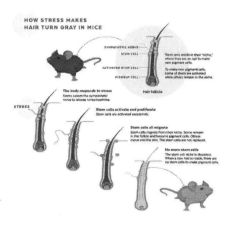

HOW STRESS MAKES
HAIR TURN GRAY IN MICE

Stress can cause high blood pressure, overeating, anxiety, fatigue, memory problems, digestive issues, insomnia, and lowered immunity.

All of those are reversible. But once your hair goes gray, there's no getting that pigment back.

WHY ARE YOU SO TIRED?

Have you been feeling more tired lately? I have and I'm hearing it a lot from clients. My 86 year old client lamented, "I'm feeling my age!"

Some stress can be positive, because it can help you to grow, to learn, and to adapt. But when stress becomes chronic, uncontrollable, unpredictable, and difficult to cope with, it begins to take a toll on your health.

Fatigue is one of the primary symptoms that can result from chronic stress and a dysfunctional stress-response system. If you're feeling highly stressed, you are more likely to suffer from not only greater fatigue, but from daytime sleepiness, poor sleep quality, and decreased sleep duration. You are also at higher risk for sleep apnea.

Which of these apply to you?

Work-related stress

Stress caused by over-commitment

Lack of social support

High demands

Lack of control

Lack of rewards

Hmmm.....I can say "all of the above." How about you?

It's important to find ways to manage our stress because we can't afford to lose precious hours of sleep.

One tactic is to control the amount of news we watch. When you're looking at bad news all day, it's going to bring you down and stress you out. Checking the news once a day is plenty.

Another approach is to put things in perspective using the "Circles of Control."

THE CIRCLES OF CONTROL

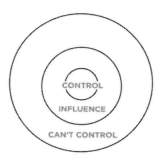

The outer circle contains things we have no influence or control over. It's the biggest one because we have no control over most things that happen in the world, like the weather, traffic, what someone thinks of us or how long the pandemic will be around.

The middle circle reflects the things we can influence, like our body composition, the atmosphere at home, and even some political agendas. While we have some influence, we don't have full control.

Where we have complete control is the inner circle. We can control what we eat, how we spend our time, who we spend our time with, and, especially, our thoughts.

Stress reduction and peace come with focus on the inner circle.

I love this wonderful play on the words from the Serenity Prayer:

"May I have the *serenity* to accept the people I cannot change, the *courage* to change the one I can, the *wisdom* to know which one that is."

REFERENCES

Top 4 Mistakes People Make When Starting A Fitness Program And How To Fix Them

1   https://tonygentilcore.com/2020/01/top-4-mistakes-beginners-make-when-starting-a-fitness-program-and- how-to-fix-them/

Why Weight Training Is Ridiculously Good For You

1   https://time.com/4803697/bodybuilding-strength-training/?utm_source=newsletter&utm_medium=e-mail&utm_campaign=time-health&utm_content=20191112

2   https://www.optimize.me/plus-one/be-fit-to-be-useful/

The Problem With "The Pause-Button Mentality"

1   https://www.precisionnutrition.com/pause-button-mentality

Captain Marvel's Got Nothing On You!

1   https://losestubbornfat.com/brie-larson-strength-training-captain-marvel/? utm_source=Dan+-John%27s+Wandering+Weights&utm_campaign=0cd93e5d12-djww243&ut-m_medium=e-mail&utm_term=0_d663067162-0cd93e5d12-36696493&goal=0_d663067162-0cd93e5d 12-36696493&mc_cid=0cd93e5d12&mc_eid=8bdfd2fc7c

Jump Squats And Silver Sneakers

1   https://www.wsj.com/articles/the-best-exercises-for-your-50s-60s-70sand-beyond-11555683513

You Don't Have To Run Far–Or Fast–To Live Longer

1   https://time.com/5720772/running-helps-you-live-longer/?utm_source=newsletter&utm_medium=e-mail&utm_campaign=time-health&utm_content=20191107

2   https://time.com/4667098/is-running-bad-for-your-knees/? utm_source=newsletter&utm_medium=e-mail&utm_campaign=time-health&utm_content=20191014

NEAT–The Non-Exercise Way To Exercise

1   *https://www.aarp.org/health/healthy-living/info-2019/non-exercise-activity-thermogenesis.html*

2   *https://www.health.harvard.edu/diet-and-weight-loss/use-the-neat-factor-nonexercise-activity-thermogenesis-to-burn-calories*

When Exercise Is An Issue Of Life Or Death

1   *https://medium.com/swlh/exercise-for-life-f6dbf174b1eb*

The TRUTH– "Core Training" Is a Meaningless Term

1   *https://medium.com/body-wisdom/the-core-strength-myth-67e3e79ac8b1*

Are Your Muscles Confused? The Part "Muscle Confusion" Plays In Your Workouts

1   *https://www.nytimes.com/2020/01/08/well/move/muscle-confusion-exercise-workouts-fitness*

Flexibility Is No Longer A Priority

1   *https://link.springer.com/article/10.1007/s40279-019-01248-w*

How Accurate Are Calorie Counts From Gym Equipment And Fitness Trackers?

1   *https://www.nutritionaction.com/daily/exercise-for-health/how-accurate-are-calorie-counts-from-gym-equipment/*

The Tyranny Of 10,000 Steps

1   *https://www.hsph.harvard.edu/news/hsph-in-the-news/10000-steps-not-magic-fitness-number/*

2   *https://www.theatlantic.com/health/archive/2016/08/the-new-exercise-mantra/495908/*

Too Old For "The Freshman 15"?

1   *https://bottomlineinc.com/life/exercise-fitness/winter-inactivity-leads-to-fast-weight-gain-muscle-loss*

The "Crossover Effect"-The Key To Working Around An Injury

1   *https://lermagazine.com/article/crossover-consequences-of-unilateral-treatments*

2   *https://doctorerinb.com/new-blog/2016/8/31/the-crossover-effect*

Exercise, Depression, And The Difference A Coach Makes

1   *https://www.nytimes.com/2019/08/21/well/move/exercise-may-boost-mood-for-women-with-depres- sion-having-a-coach-may-help.html*

Could You Forget About "Exercise" And Just Do This?

1   *https://www.amazon.com/Joy-Movement-Exercise-Happiness-Connection/dp/B07RFTPKL9/ref=sr_1_1?*

Why I Don't Believe In Weight Loss Challenges

1   https://www.otpbooks.com/product/josh-hillis-fat-loss-habits-with-dan-john/

Does Exercise Affect Weight Loss?

1   https://www.nutritionaction.com/daily/exercise-for-health/how-much-can-exercise-help-with-weight- loss/

5 Reasons Counting Calories Is Obsolete

1   https://mosaicscience.libsyn.com/why-the-calorie-is-broken-0

2   https://mosaicscience.com/story/medicine's-dirty-secret/

Any Diet Works…As Long As It Doesn't Include This One Thing

1   https://www.nytimes.com/2019/10/24/magazine/why-isnt-there-a-diet-that-works-for-everyone.html?

3 Myths About Weight Loss & Metabolism

1   https://www.ncbi.nlm.nih.gov/pmc/articles/PMC4391809/pdf/nihms676818.pdf

Portion Psychology–Use It To Your Advantage

1   https://www.nutritionaction.com/daily/how-to-diet/how-larger-portions-influence-later-choices/

2   https://www.nutritionaction.com/daily/how-to-diet/what-a-recent-study-can-tell-us-about-portion-con- trol/

The Cost Of Being Lean

1   https://www.precisionnutrition.com/cost-of-getting-lean

Flat Feet? No, You Don't Need More Arch Support

1   https://www.runnersworld.com/gear/a25750345/running-shoes-flat-feet/?

The Dark Side Of Cortisone Shots

1   https://bottomlineinc.com/health/osteoarthritis/got-hip-or-knee-arthritis-pain-a-steroid-shot-is-too- risky

So You Had An MRI Slow Down Before You Freak Out

1   https://www.instagram.com/p/B8Kp3fFlgCi/

Is It Time To Put Away The Icepack?

1   https://www.menshealth.com/fitness/a29710918/icing-sore-muscles/?

Babying Your Back Actually Delays Healing

1   https://www.health.harvard.edu/pain/babying-your-back-may-delay-healing?fbclid=IwAR2v-GUD5U-FyejIkxTPrrLwLafCxDZ2pjMqac_5FuEMEYcv3LB1jybHg6u14

Lack of Sleep Dramatically Raises Your Risk For Getting Sick

1   https://time.com/4017664/sleep-virus/?iid=sr-link1

The Best Sleeping Position Is....

1   https://pubmed.ncbi.nlm.nih.gov/6844798/

2   https://www.atsjournals.org/doi/full/10.1164/rccm.200212-1397OC

3   https://well.blogs.nytimes.com/2010/10/25/the-benefits-of-left-side-sleeping/?

3 Ways You're Affected By Sleep That You Might Not Know

1   https://www.bicycling.com/news/a26114970/cardio-fitness-heart-attack-risk/

2   https://time.com/4757521/sleep-yourself-slim/?utm_source=newsletter&utm_medium=email&utm_-

Visceral Fat– The #1 Predictor Of Disease

1   https://www.amazon.com/Fat-Chance-Beating-Against-Processed/

2   https://makeyourbodywork.com/how-to-reduce-visceral-fat/ (illustration)

Keeping Your Muscles Fit Is Tied to Better Heart Health

1   https://www.nytimes.com/2020/01/29/well/move/keeping-aging-muscles-fit-is-tied-to-better-heart-health- later

When It Comes To Depression, Exercise Can Trump Genetics

1   https://www.nytimes.com/2019/11/20/well/move/3-hours-of-exercise-a-week-may-lower-your-depres-sion-risk

2   https://onlinelibrary.wiley.com/doi/abs/10.1002/da.22967

"The Key to a Long Life Has Little to Do With 'Good Genes'"

1   https://www.wired.com/story/the-key-to-a-long-life-has-little-to-do-with-good-genes/

"Fix Your Feet"– By Changing What You Wear On Them

1   https://www.optimize.me/plus-one/how-not-to-kill-your-feet/

What You Don't Know About Shoes

1   RossiWhyShoesMakeNormalGaitImpossible.pdf

Simply Irresistible.....

1   https://www.npr.org/sections/thesalt/2019/05/16/723693839/its-not-just-salt-sugar-fat-study-finds-ultra-pro- cessed-foods-drive-weight-gain?

Instead Of An Antioxidant, Take A Placebo?

1   https://www.runnersworld.com/news/a28065471/vitamins-strength-training-study/

2   https://time.com/5375724/placebo-bill-health-problems/

3 Nutrition Sources You Can Trust

1   https://www.amazon.com/How-Eat-Your-Questions-Answered/dp/035812882X

3 Strategies For Living Longer By Becoming An Optimist

1   https://jamanetwork.com/journals/jamanetworkopen/fullarticle/

2   https://www.optimize.me/philosophers-notes/golden-rules-for-everyday-life-omraam-mikhael-aivanhov/

Celebrate! It'll Make You Happier!

1   https://www.bluezones.com/2019/12/science-says-celebrating-holidays-could-make-you-happier/

2   https://journals.plos.org/plosone/article?id=10.1371/journal.pone.0073791

3   https://www.sciencedirect.com/science/article/abs/pii/S0272494489800106

Stress Really Can Give You Gray Hair

1   https://newsinhealth.nih.gov/2020/04/how-stress-causes-gray-hair

ABOUT THE AUTHOR

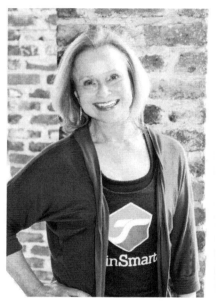

Susan graduated with a B.S. degree from Auburn University and began her fitness career in 1985, teaching group fitness classes for Executive Fitness at the US Geological Survey in Reston, VA. She was gold certified as a personal trainer by the American Council on Exercise in 1990. In 1998, she received her Level I Resistance Training Specialist certification and became the only certified ChiWalking/ChiRunning instructor in the Southeast in 2007. In 2011, she was awarded the Corrective Exercise Specialist certification from the National Association of Sports Medicine, and corrective exercise has become her specialty.

After 27 years in the fitness industry, including 20 years at the Birmingham Jewish Community Center, as both a personal trainer and ultimately the personal training coordinator, Susan opened **TrainSmarter** in 2014. She completed multiple TRX qualifications, including the highest TRX certification, TRX TEAM. In an effort to reach more people, she became NCFI Corporate Fitness Specialist certified in 2016 and Online Training Specialist certified in 2019.

Susan's specialties include corrective exercise, strength training, gait analysis and running technique, online training, corporate wellness, TRX training and mentoring fitness professionals.

Made in the USA
Columbia, SC
25 April 2021

36350221R00115